A LETTER FROM DIANA DEGETTE, FIRST CONGRESSIONAL DISTRICT, COLORADO

OUR food safety system is a woefully under-funded system designed during the latter half of the twentieth century that has failed to adapt to the twenty-first century marketplace. Recall after recall has sounded the alarm that our food safety system in America is broken. No one knows this as well as the Moore family.

The tale Kip Moore tells in this book is a heartbreaking one—a father committed to his young son, Chance, who became sickened from contaminated food. While tragic, Kip and Chance's story is a solemn reminder to us all of the thousands who fell sick or who died as a result of faulty gaps and holes in our nation's food safety system. Chance's second chance is a story of the lucky ones. Kip has done a remarkable job of putting a real face on this scourge—transporting readers to his son's bedside as he and his wife huddle with their ailing child. His book will tug your emotions, and you will put it down with a human understanding of this problem.

I first met Kip Moore two years ago when he participated in a food safety discussion I hosted in Colorado. Kip was just beginning his crusade against food safety regulations that would culminate in the publishing of this book, and I was continuing my efforts to move Congress with the same sense of urgency to reform the system. Meeting Kip and seeing first-hand the intense dedication he was bringing to the issue was a reinvigorating experience for me, and I returned to Congress with yet another concrete example of why this fight was necessary. The circumstances that became the impetus for this book are sad, and the picture it paints of our food safety infrastructure is grave. But the story it tells is also uplifting and hopeful—the tale of a young boy's indomitable will to survive and a family determined to ensure its son's safety.

For Kip, his son, and families everywhere, Congress is committed to comprehensive food safety reform, and we will do it. We will not only do it on behalf of Chance, but also for the children and their parents everywhere our food safety system failed to protect.

—**Diana DeGette,**
First Congressional District, Colorado

Second Chance

*The Story of a Father's Faith,
a Mother's Strength,
and a Child's Will to Live*

Kip Moore

Second Chance Publishing LLC
Golden, Colorado

First printing 2010

ISBN 978-0-9841673-5-7
LCCN 2009907309

DEDICATION

To our children: Shannon, TJ, Loryn, and Chance. You are the light of our lives and the best part of us.

Love,
Dad and Mom

CONTENTS

ACKNOWLEDGMENTS

THIS book would not be complete without the people who were instrumental in its creation. I thank all the doctors and nurses at The Children's Hospital who were involved in Chance's care. They include Dr. Brian Stenga, who taught me a new meaning for the game Asteroids; Dr. Kelly Fitzgerald, who saved Chance's life; and nurse Molly Oedkoven, who showed so much compassion toward us. Without your dedication and help, Chance would not be with us today. I would also like to thank Chance's pediatrician, Dr. Nikki Bacon. Dr. Bacon, we did not stop for anything.

Thanks to my close friends: Willy, Andy, Coov, and Nitch. Thank you for all of your support throughout this difficult time and for your loyal friendship over the years. You all define what the word friendship truly means. A special thanks to my dear friend Amy Cleavinger who received a number of panicked phone calls from me. I'll never be able to repay you for everything that you did for us during this trying time.

A heartfelt thank you goes to my parents, Al and Connie Moore, who gave up a month of their lives in Kansas to stay at our home in Denver. Thanks also to Marti's sister Heather who kept our lives going by taking care of our household for a week. Thanks to my sister Cristen Tilden; my cousin Brad Johnson; our dear friends Patti and Carl; Chance's loving babysitter, Peggy; and Marti's friends, coworkers, and sister Beth for their love, prayers, and support. Marti and I are lucky to have such loving friends and family.

Thanks to Kelly Jo Eldredge and Eric Mott, who assisted me with the writing of this book. Your skillful words helped me to make this project possible.

Finally, I would like to thank God and all of those who prayed for Chance during this challenging time. This book would not have been possible without prayer.

FOREWORD BY
CONGRESSWOMAN LYNN JENKINS, TOPEKA, KS

I'VE known Kip and the Moore family for over fifteen years, and my favorite word to describe them is *inspiring*. They live their lives with joy; they nurture each other with love; and they have a unique way of encouraging those around them. My life is better because of my friendship with Kip and his family, and I am honored that he asked me to contribute the foreword to his first book.

I sought Kip's advice when I initially thought about going into politics, because I was unsure about taking the plunge into government service. When I told Kip about my aspirations to serve the people of Kansas his response was honest and immediate. He told me without reservation that I should do it, and that he always felt it was important to chase your dreams.

"Lynn, if you really pour your heart into running for office, I think you would be terrific." Kip told me. "You're a great listener, and I know you would always put your constituents ahead of any personal agenda."

That is Kip. He's positive, encouraging, and above all inspiring.

I was heartbroken when I discovered Kip and Marti's son Chance contracted E. coli three years ago. As a mother, my whole world revolves around my children, Hayden and Hayley. I could hardly imagine what the Moore family must have gone through during those tense days in the hospital. Our family did our best to stay in touch with Kip and Marti during that time. We closely followed the news updates on The Children's Hospital care page website, and our thoughts and prayers were with them always. Their journey was a difficult one, and I was once again inspired by the strength, courage, and faith this family exhibited. Their love for Chance was fierce, and their support of him was extraordinary.

After a month of uncertainty, we were elated when we heard Chance was coming home from the hospital, once again a healthy and vibrant little boy. I wish Chance the best for a long and healthy life. We are all "cheating" for Chance, and I look forward to watching him follow his dreams as he grows into adulthood.

I am also so very proud of Kip for having the courage to share his story. I believe this book will have a strong impact on parents and families everywhere. One of my greatest fears is the possibility of losing a child to an unforeseen illness like E. coli. Chance survived, and this book is a wonderful testament to the resilience of a brave little boy and the constant vigilance of an exceptional family.

If you are in need of hope, if you could use a dose of inspiration, I highly recommend *Second Chance*.

—Congresswoman Lynn Jenkins
Topeka, Kansas 2009

PROLOGUE

PARENTS need the courage to hope. We need the strength to fight on our children's behalf in their time of need. How can young children who are sick know what is happening to them? They do not understand the concept of a mortal illness. They can only feel the physical pain of their afflictions and experience the fear of the moment. We parents experience pain and fear of a different kind: deep-rooted empathy for our offspring, the emotional pain of impending separation…dreading the unbearable possibility of a lifetime's potential to be denied.

Parents need the strength to face that dread and still support our sons and daughters at all costs—keeping them safe is our sacred task. We cannot feel our children's hurts for them, as much as we wish we could. But hope gives us the strength to have compassion for our children and assure them that they are not alone, and that their lifeline is intact.

I needed hope.

THE small, windowless waiting room outside the pediatric intensive care unit offered no sanctuary, and the 1970s décor offered no comfort. I sat with my wife, Marti, on the edge of the single couch in that confining, prickly room; and held her, numbed, dazed, and frightened. We felt like we had been hit by a freight train. Just three hours before, our little boy stopped breathing and required forty-five minutes of resuscitation to come back—he came back! Now, he was in intensive care.

My courage and strength were waning; I knew my job was to protect my son but I no longer knew how. A week without sleep, my own illness, deep feelings of guilt, and the wild careening from one crisis to another had left me bereft of the hope I needed to provide strength for my son and my family. Even the adrenaline of the latest crisis was not enough to sustain me for long. We were drained. Where would we find the courage now to brace ourselves so that we could sustain him? Where would we find the wisdom to continue to make life and death decisions for our son?

An intensive care nurse walked in to the room. I wish I could remember her name, but I don't. As I rose to meet her, I had one dreadful question on my mind. For the second time since this nightmare started I asked this question, and this time I would not be denied: "Is my son going to die?"

My wife and I will never forget what happened next; we will never forget the answer we received. Without flinching the nurse looked at me in the eye and said, "We do *not* let kids die...."

How could she make such an audacious guarantee? She could not. My son was near death, and the three of us knew it. But that wise nurse knew what we needed most at that moment: the courage to sustain ourselves during our difficult trial. There was a truth to her words that struck deeper than their literal meaning. Her words contained hope.

It worked. I woke up with a rush and knew from then on we could find the strength to fight together with our son in his battle for his life. He was ours and we were his, and we would not leave his side or give up. We loved him. The nurse's bold words became my mantra from then on:

We do not let kids die....

CHAPTER 1

Introducing Chance

"DAD? Dad! Who are you cheating for?"

I love to watch sports on television, especially if my five-year-old son joins me. He sits close to me on the couch so I can put my arm around him. Sometimes we eat cookies or chips together; sometimes we just watch. I always put my arm around him—close, safe…adored. He is my son Chance. This is his story.

It's hard not to crack a smile or chuckle when I look down into his earnest blue eyes after he asks me that question. Harder yet when I notice his unruly sandy-brown hair—he has a cowlick that makes it impossible to comb. Somewhere along the line he misplaced the word "cheating" for "rooting," and it's stuck ever since. He'll learn the proper word soon enough. For now, I find his phraseology so endearing I refuse to correct it. It makes my heart constrict with love for him.

After I tell him which team I am rooting for—usually the Kansas Jayhawks—he will return his gaze to the television. This is our precious time together, time to bond as father and son. If no game is on, we'll watch *American Idol* or *Dancing with the Stars*. He'll probably be a singing and dancing basketball star when he grows up.

When he's finished with his snack he will suck his thumb and continue to watch TV with his head resting on my shoulder. I know most parents try to break their kids' thumb-sucking habit, but I can't force myself to do so with Chance. To me, his thumb sucking is a triumph of life and spirit.

There was a time once when Chance was so sick that he didn't have the strength or will to do anything, including suck his thumb. So let him do it now! It reminds me that he is alive. His crooked teeth can be fixed but his kidneys cannot, and his life is irreplaceable. He is my hero and the bravest boy I know, and I want to tell you his story.

Let me tell you Chance's story for his sake, so that he will always know how special and loved he is. In the future he can read this and appreciate the precious and fragile nature of life. Let me tell you his story for my sake so that I will never forget it—or take my son for granted. Perhaps in the telling I will also heal myself and can lay aside the feelings of fear and guilt I carry to this day. This story is for us.

I want to tell you his story for the sake of all parents who may face a situation in the future where their child's life is threatened with illness or injury. You can find the strength to fight for them no matter how dark the days and nights become. Strength can come from surprising places if you keep your hearts and minds open to all its possible sources. This story is for the parents of sick children.

Let's celebrate Chance's story together! There were so many heroic people involved in his care to whom I owe a debt of thanks. I want to celebrate and honor them: doctors, nurses, technicians, and a very special hospital, The Children's Hospital of Denver. In humble gratitude, this story is for them.

Finally, there was a spiritual aspect of Chance's recovery. This book is for those who believe, or need to believe, that physical healing cannot always be explained through medicine or science. Events I can't comprehend occurred that convinced me that God had his hand on my son the entire time he was ill. Events occurred that inspired me to pray over him each night saying, "God, please continue to keep him safe from harm." This story is for those yearning to learn the power of prayer.

My wife and I named Chance in honor of the second chance she and I were given to find true love and happiness with each other. I'm doubly proud of his name now that it represents his second chance on life. Watching TV on the couch with him is a sacred ritual for me that I hope we never forsake—our father and son time.

"Who are you cheating for, Dad?"

I'm cheating for you, son.

CHAPTER 2

Mount Rushmore

THE brightly colored collection of state flags matched my family's cheerful mood that day, July 29, 2005. A paved walkway flanked by rows of square, stone pillars stretched before us. Each pillar supported four flagpoles, one on each side. The colorful archway formed by the flags beckoned us to move forward to view the national monument beyond. They offered a striking contrast to the gray stone faces of George, Thomas, Teddy, and Abe rising high above the Avenue of Flags.

We stopped there and posed for some pictures. We tried to arrange ourselves in the same stately manner as our founding fathers above us. The Mount Rush-Moores—we deserved to be on television. Luckily for us, our moment of fame was at hand! A reporter with cameraman in tow approached us and asked us for an interview.

The faces of the presidents gleamed that weekend as the memorial celebrated its recent restoration. Crews had spent months power washing the lichens off the granite faces—and from inside the nostrils—of four of our most revered commanders-in-chief. Television teams wanted to capture the festivities on tape.

"Hello. Would you and your family like to do a television interview?" the reporter asked.

"Sure!" I replied, pushing my family forward and stepping out of the way. I had my reasons for staying off-camera, but I mostly wanted this to be their moment.

I smiled as I watched the reporter arrange the children in front of Marti. They looked nervous, but I could tell they were having fun. Their excitement had been evident ever since we saw the huge monument rise above the pine trees as we drove up the winding road to the memorial. I was proud of them all and excited they had this opportunity to be on television.

"Where are you from?" the reporter asked Marti.

"Denver, Colorado," she replied.

Excellent! Marti is camera shy, so I was pleased that she kept her composure.

"Did you come for the restoration opening?"

"Honestly, no. We didn't know that was happening today. We just wanted the kids to see Mount Rushmore."

True enough. We made the seven-hour car trip from Denver the day before to attend the vow renewals of one of Marti's high school friends. Marti grew up in South Dakota, but had not seen the monument for quite some time. I had not seen it since age ten. We felt that we could not pass up this chance to show the kids this famous site.

The reporter turned his attention to my son TJ. "So, what do you think of Mount Rushmore?"

"It's really big," TJ said quietly.

Brilliant! TJ, my son from my first marriage, was eleven that summer, and getting ready for the fall competitive soccer season. I am a sports nut so I couldn't wait to attend his upcoming matches.

Next came Loryn's turn, my stepdaughter. The eight-year-old was a swimmer and spent a lot of her summertime in the pool. Loryn, the budding actor, loved to make up shows and perform them for us. This was her chance to get noticed.

"How about you? What do you think?"

She replied with the grace of a future actor. "It's beautiful."

Awesome! They were in rare form, and full of useful information.

Finally, Chance's turn came. He represented our last opportunity to impress the nation with the Moore family wit and wisdom. I couldn't wait to hear what our eighteen-month-old son was going to say. One of his famous "Chance-isms" was about to be captured on tape, I hoped. My son, wearing a cute purple shirt, jean shorts, and little black sandals, was about to stun the world.

"Hey little guy, what do you think?"

Chance promptly stuck his thumb in his mouth and hid coyly behind Marti, grabbing her leg—so much for grand pronouncements.

The reporter laughed out loud. "There you have it, three approvals on the restoration and one undecided."

I couldn't wait to tell my daughter, Shannon, about this. She couldn't make the trip because she was attending a dance camp with her Golden High School dance team members. We had a blended family; we had a loving family. I was very proud that day. You can't take family and happiness for granted.

A recent scare served to increase my gratitude that day even more. Less than two weeks before our South Dakota trip we faced the frightful possibility of losing our home. The North Table Mountain wildfire near Golden, Colorado came dangerously close to our subdivision. Authorities asked us to prepare to evacuate, and we nearly did. I moved piles of furniture and belongings into our driveway and even got as far as loading them into our van. Chance helped as much as a little tike could. Our neighbors and friends around us made the same hurried preparations as we did.

Chance was on tape that day, too. Marti has a friend who is a reporter with the local NBC affiliate. That friend asked to interview Marti on camera regarding the fire, but she got shy at the last minute and substituted me. That's part of the reason I ducked out of the Mount Rushmore taping—to get her back!

When my interview ran on the ten o'clock news that night, the station included footage of Chance sitting in our van with our possessions. Another clip showed him standing in our front yard, sucking his thumb of course.

No, you can't take a blessed life for granted. The fire did not touch our house or the neighborhood that day. That allowed us to take our vacation to the Black Hills worry-free, thankful that we had averted a potentially life-changing situation. We were in South Dakota celebrating the renewal vows of our good friends, and evidently, the restoration of Mount Rushmore. Most importantly, we were celebrating family, as we did at all times—Marti, Shannon, TJ, Loryn, Chance, and me. Life was good.

We raced back to our hotel room to watch the Mount Rush-Moores on the evening news.

CHAPTER 3

A Father's Choices

"I DON'T want to alarm you, but I want you to drive directly to The Children's Hospital from my office. Don't stop anywhere."

I most certainly was alarmed—terrified, in fact. Our idyllic family vacation had turned into a nightmare in just a few confusing days. How could I not be alarmed? Chance's pediatrician had just told us to drive him to one of Denver's premier hospitals *without stopping anywhere.* How did it come to this?

Dr. Bacon typically possessed a calm, businesslike manner when she examined Chance, but that day was different. She had an edge to her mannerisms that set me on alert. The serious tone of her voice frightened me more than her words, and I saw her eyes narrow with concern. But still, she was calm. *I don't want to alarm you.* That phrase achieved the opposite.

Dr. Bacon explained to us that Chance's relentless diarrhea could be from either a viral or bacterial infection. I heard the term E. coli for the first time and asked Dr. Bacon to explain what she meant. E. coli is an intestinal bacterium that can cause a serious infection when ingested—like from a piece of uncooked meat, she said. Then, I confessed that I had been sick all week with similar symptoms, as sick as I had ever been, in fact. That did it! *Drive directly to The Children's Hospital!*

My heart felt like it was in my stomach by the time we reached our minivan; my movements felt slow and exaggerated. Marti and I loaded our miserable, whimpering boy into his car seat in silence and drove into the unknown. *Where is The Children's Hospital?*

Marti and I exchanged brief words regarding driving directions, and then resumed our silent journey. We both felt consumed by our own fearful thoughts. I was starting to panic by then and backtracking in my mind trying to guess what could have happened during the last few days to cause this dreadful situation. A surging wave of helplessness began to overcome me.

We drove in silence underneath gray, wet skies. My unseeing eyes barely noticed the roads we traveled in that twenty-minute journey to the hospital. We were lucky we didn't get into a car accident on the way. We had witnessed a car accident on our recent vacation: the image of that vehicle wrapped around a telephone pole was still fresh in my mind.

We had a wreck of a different sort in progress. My precious son's health was deteriorating rapidly, and I had to get him to a hospital *without stopping*. How did it come to this?

By the time we reached the Children's emergency room entrance, my fear and dread had intensified. I dropped Marti and Chance off and watched them disappear through the hospital doors. I could not stand to be separated from them, so I parked the car as quickly as I could.

When I cut the ignition, though, I paused. Anger and guilt began to rise up within me. I thought, *What kind of father am I?*

Tears moistened my eyes as I began to berate myself, and I gripped the car's steering wheel until my knuckles turned white. My mind was bubbling with questions of self-doubt: Why did I ignore Chance's bloody diarrhea so long? What if his life was now at risk due to my delays? Why didn't I call Marti sooner?

I was Chance's father. That small child depended on me to make decisions each day to protect him. That was my job. What if I had made different choices in the past four days? Would we be in a different situation?

I tried to compose myself as best as I could. I wanted to regain control before I entered the hospital so I wouldn't be a basket case. I needed to have the calmness to make better choices from here on out. Scenes from the previous days kept replaying in my head, however; I couldn't stop them.

Oh, god! How did it come to this?

MONDAY morning, August 1, began a week that we thought would be like any other. We had just completed a joyous weekend vacation to South Dakota. The Table Mountain wildfire was receding into our memories. We had every expectation that this week would be a continuation of our rich, happy journey together as a family. Little did we know that we were about to take a radical detour. Marti drove to work and took Chance with her, to drop off at daycare. *Just another day, right?*

You know when you wake up in the morning and you feel achy and blah, not sure whether you'll be able to get out of bed, let alone make it through the day? I awoke Monday morning wishing I felt that good. Flu-like symptoms bothered me, but I couldn't tell for sure what was causing them. I simply told Marti that I felt "out of sorts."

In typical male fashion, I'm slow to admit that something is wrong with me and even slower to visit a doctor. Monday was different, however. Whatever illness I had progressed so rapidly,

I couldn't wait to see my doctor by two o'clock in the afternoon. They could not do much for me—took some blood; told me I had food poisoning, or something like that; I was a healthy adult…just wait it out—blah, blah, blah. However, while at the doctor's office, I discovered the fastest way to find yourself hooked up to an EKG machine is to faint in the presence of your nurse. I had gone well beyond "out of sorts," but I returned home.

Convinced I was feeling as sick as I had ever been, I spent that evening in bed, padding my body with as many pillows as I could find. I could not stand to be touched anywhere. My diarrhea began that evening, and it lasted for ten days. Ten of the most crucial days of my life followed, and I was saddled with a bad case of diarrhea and no appetite.

Chance vomited for the first time at ten o'clock that night.

At that time, I worked for myself as an investment consultant out of our house. I decided that I needed to keep Chance at home with me the next day. He had had a rough time overnight. Marti spent the night with him; they slept together in our guest bedroom. He vomited several times, but it ended by eight o'clock Tuesday morning. Chance looked so lethargic and puny to me, and I took care of him as best I could. I was still viciously ill, of course. Parents can take a day off from work, but you can't stop caring for your children no matter what you feel like. Investment consultants can call in sick, but fathers cannot.

After Marti returned home from work that evening, I sent her out again to get milkshakes for Chance and me. I was going on forty-eight hours without significant food or drink. Marti was so intent on her milkshake mission that she got a speeding ticket on the way home. It wasn't that urgent; we were hungry but we weren't dying, or so I thought. In spite of her efforts, I couldn't keep my milkshake down and neither could Chance.

Later that night, we heard Chance crying over his baby monitor. Marti investigated and found him literally swimming in a pool of diarrhea in his crib. She picked him up by the armpits and dunked him in the bathtub to clean him up. She slept with him in the guest bedroom again.

On Wednesday, Marti left Chance and me home together for a second day. We passed the day much as we did the previous one. Neither of us felt well, but we were surviving. At one o'clock in the afternoon, however, Chance passed his first bloody stool. Unfortunately, I shrugged it off. I thought it was just a result of all the irritation he must have been experiencing. I could relate to that.

A few hours later, when changing Chance's diaper again, I noticed an even bigger and bloodier stool. That got my attention, so I drove my son from our home in Golden to a nearby urgent care center in the Denver suburb of Lakewood.

Once there, the nurses escorted us to a large, intimidating, and cold room. Chance's white skin matched the pale lighting of that uninviting place. I shivered. The medical professionals quickly determined Chance was severely dehydrated—not surprising considering the level of vomiting and diarrhea he had been experiencing. They prescribed an IV to replace his lost fluids.

Watching your child get poked with an IV needle has to be one of the hardest things for a parent to do. I couldn't look. I had to turn my back; I should have stepped out of the room. I gritted my teeth and tensed upon on hearing Chance scream and cry with pain and fear. His arm was wrapped in so much protective gauze when it was over that it looked like it belonged on the Michelin Man. Forty-five minutes later, Chance had received his first bolus of IV fluid.

In spite of these events, I still felt nothing was seriously wrong. Just the flu. I had it, too. What the doctor told me next caused me to rethink my diagnosis.

"I don't want to alarm you, but we've contacted Lutheran Hospital. I think you should take Chance there. He's not perking up as much as we would like—let them do a thorough examination."

I don't want to alarm you. Great.

I called Marti at that point, interrupting her dinner business meeting. I could barely get the words out, because the first pangs of guilt started to creep into my gut for ignoring that initial bloody stool. Our child was sick, we were at urgent care, and now we had to go to the hospital. Marti was calm but concerned, and she agreed to cut her dinner short and meet us there.

Once we arrived at Lutheran Hospital's emergency department, we were ushered into another exam room. This one was much smaller than the first but equally uninviting. Of course another IV was required, but having learned my lesson, I stepped outside when the technicians stuck Chance's arm. Marti stayed and held his hand.

We tried everything we could think of to distract Chance while he received his second bolus of IV fluid of the day: Popsicles, television, and movies. His diarrhea came twice an hour and the doctors wanted to take a sample, but that was nearly impossible because it was so runny.

Chance tolerated the infusion of fluids and seemed perkier to me. After four hours of treatment, at one o'clock in the morning, the Lutheran staff suggested that we go home. They asked us to contact our pediatrician the following day for the results of Chance's tests and warned us to keep him hydrated. We went home. None of us got any sleep; Chance and I both continued to be extremely sick.

A COLD front passed over Denver and its suburbs that night. We could feel the chill in the air when we returned from Lutheran hospital in the early morning hours of Thursday, August 4. The weather was extremely cold for August in Colorado. It was doubly noticeable because the temperature had dropped thirty degrees from Wednesday.

Marti decided to stay home that cold, rainy day and take her conference calls there. By nine thirty, I knew Chance was not well. He looked even paler, and very lethargic. Suppressing my urge to panic as best I could, I picked him up, entered Marti's office, and told her we needed to see a doctor. *Now.*

We got in the car and drove to Dr. Bacon's office. Rain clouds were gathering outside as we drove, the same way they gathered in our lives in the form of our son's darkly deteriorating health. From there we drove straight to The Children's Hospital, without stopping.

Marti and Chance would not return home for nearly a month.

CHAPTER 4

The Children's Hospital

KIDS are smart—even very sick ones. Chance knew well by then what getting an IV meant and saw his third one coming from a mile away. Marti and I held his arms and legs down while the nurse placed the needle in his poor little arm. For a few excruciating minutes, I thought Chance's piercing screams would cause me to go deaf. Then finally the IV was in place and began dripping vital, life-sustaining fluid into my precious boy's body.

We were now at The Children's Hospital, in yet another cold examining room. Despite his fever of 101 degrees and heart rate of 146 beats per minute, Chance was shivering due to the infusion of fluids, so we placed a blanket over him and waited…and waited. Marti tirelessly changed his diaper every thirty minutes. She was unbelievable.

Nothing feels longer than the period of time waiting for a decision to be made while in the emergency room with a sick child. We vainly tried to get Chance to drink some Gatorade, but he would not take it. The only fluids he received were from his IV line. Four hours felt like four days to us. Then, around six o'clock in the evening, the doctors told us of their decision to admit Chance to the hospital.

I was relieved. I recovered from my angry moment in the parking lot but feelings of guilt still assailed me, and the stress of making uninformed decisions was beginning to pile up. My shoulders felt lighter when I heard the doctor say he was admitting Chance. Now, I thought, I could leave the decisions to the professionals. We were safe, now, and I was off the hook.

The hospital staff had trouble finding a room for us on that busy night at The Children's Hospital. We eventually landed in a fourth-floor room with another child who was soon moved out. We were then alone, and Chance found himself in a large bed hooked up to a heart monitor.

The room's accommodations for parents weren't the best, but the bed was quite large. So Marti decided the best thing she could do to comfort him was to climb in bed with him. She still bore the brunt of his onslaught of required diaper changes. She could barely keep up, so the friendly, comforting staff began to help; they were real heroes, helping us like that. It was a horrific sight to witness so many bloody diapers. I couldn't bear to watch my son's life oozing away like that and had to step outside.

The nurses began taking blood samples from Chance for analysis. Every two hours they pricked his body with needles. By then he barely noticed them because he was too lethargic. Chance's doctor, Dr. Stanga, visited us next. He explained to us that he would be watching Chance for the next forty-eight hours, and that his condition had not been diagnosed. I asked him if Chance had E. coli, but he replied that test results had not confirmed that yet. I had an inkling that's what he was thinking, though.

Dr. Stanga told us it was too soon to prescribe antibiotics; besides, they could possibly do more harm than good at that point. He said the best we could do that first night was to offer supportive care and deal with any situation that might arise. With that, he left, assuring us that he was on call and could return at a moment's notice if necessary.

We braced ourselves for a long night.

A long night, indeed. Marti and I hoped that Chance would find some rest, but it was not to be. He began experiencing severe stomach pains and cramps associated with his stools. By one o'clock Friday morning the decision was made to take some abdominal images to check for an intestinal blockage. When the nurses came to take Chance for his CT scan, he screamed loudly. He did not want to be separated from Marti. That was so hard on her, too. She wavered a little, and I did my best to console her.

While Chance was out of the room, I encouraged Marti to eat to regain her strength. She had spent several hours in Chance's bed by that point without moving. She had no appetite but forced some food down anyway. She was equally concerned for me. I was still battling my own intestinal infection and could not eat, either. We were quite the pair. We were in sad shape, but we had each other. For Chance's sake, we agreed to focus on him instead of ourselves.

Forty-five minutes later Chance returned to his room. Chance's intestines were not blocked but severely inflamed. We resumed our sleepless vigil, and Marti took up position with Chance in his bed once more. The schedule of blood draws resumed, too. Nurses were already running out of new places to poke him—arms, legs, fingers, toes—they had all been used. By dawn Chance looked like a pincushion.

Morning came and questions about Chance's condition remained unanswered. E. coli? Flu? Some other form of food poisoning? What was wrong with our child?

Our endless night was over, but our stay at The Children's Hospital had just begun.

In a few short days my son had been reduced to a shell of his former self. Normally he had such a bubbly, active personality. However, after less than twenty-four hours in the hospital, he could only lay lifeless and unresponsive in Marti's arms. He no longer sucked his thumb.

I had visions of Chance's morning ritual at our house. He always had such a big, beautiful smile for me when I came downstairs for breakfast, and his voice would sing out as he sat in his high chair. He would say, "Hi, Daddy. I'm eating!" That always made me laugh.

I missed my son.

CHAPTER 5

Exploding Asteroids

WE completed our first twenty-four hours at The Children's Hospital much the same way we started them: confused, scared, and no closer to learning what was wrong with Chance or what caused his condition. Marti and I had not slept since we arrived. We began to pay a heavy emotional and physical toll for being awake for so long.

Chance's routine of frequent diarrhea and painful sticks for blood work continued relentlessly. All three of us were exhausted. That afternoon, Dr. Stanga visited us in Chance's room to discuss our case. With the exception of the previous night's X-ray, this was the first time Marti left Chance's side. We were eager and hopeful to finally learn what made him so ill.

Dr. Stanga sat the both of us down and explained our son's diagnosis to us. He gave us a lot of information that was hard to comprehend with minds fogged by sleeplessness and worry. Even though Chance's stool cultures had not yet revealed an E. coli infection, Dr. Stanga felt that his symptoms and blood tests suggested *hemolytic-uremic syndrome*, or HUS.

Hemolytic-uremic syndrome is a serious condition caused by toxins in the bloodstream released by the bacterium, E. coli.

"Hemolytic" means a red blood cell-destroying process; while "uremic" refers to a process involving the buildup of wastes in the blood due to failure of the kidneys. E. coli is *Escherichia coli*, a common bacterium found in the lower intestines of most mammals, including people. However, a dangerous strain of E. coli called O157:H7 can cause serious health consequences when ingested by children, the elderly, or people who are already ill. Children are the most vulnerable.

In a young child, HUS begins after gastroenteritis, an inflammation of the intestines, causes a bout with bloody diarrhea that releases the E. coli toxins, called *verotoxins*, into the bloodstream. These toxic chemicals adhere to and damage the lining of the blood vessels, causing a severe inflammatory reaction all over the body. Platelets, the tiny cells that help blood to clot, stick to the inflamed vessel walls and create a mesh that shears apart the much larger red blood cells. Then the insidious downward spiral begins.

This abnormal red blood cell destruction can be catastrophic to a patient's kidneys. They are small enough to enter the filtering areas of the kidneys but too big to pass into the urine. The kidneys get clogged and begin to shut down. This is called *acute renal failure*, and it is a life-threatening situation.

In addition to the vomiting and diarrhea, most children get pale, irritable, and tired with HUS because of anemia. Sometimes blood transfusions are required to combat the loss of so many red blood cells. Many children develop kidney failure, and the worst cases require dialysis to support life.

Even after hearing Dr. Stanga's diagnosis and explanation, neither Marti nor I clearly understood what was happening or how serious Chance's condition really was. The information was swimming upstream against the sleep deprivation. I spoke first.

"How did Chance get this?"

"You can get an infection of this nature in various ways, but the most common one is through something you and Chance ate—undercooked beef, maybe," he replied.

We then discussed where we might have eaten such a meal. We weren't sure, but we narrowed it down to a breakfast we had in South Dakota. Whatever it was caused Chance and I to become really sick, Marti just a little, and the other kids, TJ and Loryn, not at all.

I still wasn't sure I was getting the whole picture, however, so I asked Dr. Stanga to repeat his definition in simpler terms.

"Kip, did you play the video game, Asteroids, growing up?"

I blinked and wondered what his question meant. I told Dr. Stanga that yes, I had. He said shooting the asteroids cause pieces of rock to sheer off, making more flying rocks. He explained that platelets inappropriately attaching to Chance's blood vessel walls were shearing off pieces of red cells, just like in the game. These fragments clog up the filtering apparatus of the kidneys, and they could shut down as a result.

The analogy helped me, but then a dreaded question entered my head—the question every parent of a seriously ill child thinks but is afraid to speak. I couldn't keep the question silent anymore, so I blurted, "Is Chance going to die?"

Next to me, Marti began to cry.

Dr. Stanga gave me a stern look, told me I was asking good questions, but said I had to stop "scaring your wife."

The next forty-eight hours were crucial, according to Dr. Stanga. He said he would order Chance to be catheterized so that he could monitor his urine output. He prepared us as best he could for the very real possibility of kidney failure and prescribed a drug immediately that would inhibit platelets from sticking in Chance's blood vessels.

Our doctor closed the conversation by saying we should not fight this presumptive E. coli infection with antibiotics. If we suddenly killed all the bacteria, more toxins would be released and the situation could worsen exponentially. The best we could do, in his opinion, was play defense. This meant supporting Chance the best we could by dealing with conditions as they arose. Aggressive treatments such as blood transfusions and antibiotics would just add more fuel to the fire inside my son's body. Too many asteroids were flying around his bloodstream already.

Dr. Stanga said goodbye and left the room. Marti and I were devastated; we held each other and cried openly. We returned to our son's bedside and held his hand, forcing ourselves to muster the courage to tell him everything was going to be okay. It was so hard to do.

As Marti resumed her vigil at Chance's side, I stepped out of the room. I began the grim process of contacting family members to tell them the serious news. I found myself in the fourth-floor waiting area, staring blankly at the walls; I could barely comprehend what was happening to us. I was numb.

Breakfast in South Dakota—why couldn't we have all ordered the pancakes?

HEARING Chance's diagnosis from Dr. Stanga and calling relatives with the news was a bleak, exhausting task. I barely understood the clinical picture myself, but I had to repeat it over and over again to them over the phone. The experience of making those calls deepened my guilt even further. I couldn't shake the irrational thought that it was my fault Chance fell sick, because of something I knowingly gave him to eat. I needed a refuge, a place to clear my head, so I asked for directions to the hospital's chapel.

The intimate room on the first floor with the ornate wooden doors reminded me of a Catholic church, though on a much smaller scale. I sat in a wooden pew on the right side—the aisle seat of the second row—and I prayed. I prayed with my head bowed and held in my hands; I prayed like I have never prayed before. I asked God to give Chance the strength to fight this illness. I prayed for Marti and me to be strong also and to have the wisdom to make the correct decisions for Chance's care.

I prayed and prayed, for what seemed like hours. In addition to God, I prayed to the spirits of every deceased relative I could think of for their guidance and strength, too. I prayed to Grandpa Ray, who came to all my youth sports games, and I prayed to Grandma Ginnie, who never learned to drive but made awesome homemade meals. I prayed to Gran Gran, who taught my sister and me to love Icees at the 7-Eleven. Finally, I prayed to Grandma Rossie, the special one. I prayed to them all.

I even prayed to the spirit of my ex father-in-law—TJ and Shannon's Grandpa Larry.

You never know.

Time stood still for me as I prayed that afternoon, Friday, August 5. Then... *what was that?* I looked up at the stained glass window, the only source of light in the dim room. I don't remember what scene the window depicted, only that the splash of color caught my attention, a splash of color that morphed into something else. What was that? I felt cold...a chill...goosebumps?

A vision was placed before my eyes, or was it my imagination? I couldn't tell. I saw myself holding Chance in the doorway of his hospital room. He wore his jean shorts and sandals, and his blue shirt with the multi-colored stripes across the chest. We were alone in the hospital; no one else could be seen. Quietly, we walked down the hallway, in the slow, silent walk of a man in a dream.

Tendrils of fog swirled around my feet, and a mist hovered over my vision. I couldn't see where I was going but I continued on, anyway. I saw Chance's face clearly, though, right next to me. He wore his famous mischievous grin—I would have recognized it anywhere. Eventually, before me I saw a light getting brighter with each step. The shape of the emergency room doors rose up before me.

I paused there, uncertain, and looked back into the misty corridor. Tears formed in my eyes as I stood there. I then heard Chance's voice in my ear saying, "Come on, Dad! Let's go!"

The tears flowed stronger, and I replied, "Yes! Let's go!" We stepped out of the sliding emergency room doors and into the bright light of the outside world: clear, cloudless, and full of color. My heart soared as we left the threshold of the building and I felt light enough that I could fly.

Chance was released from the hospital! He was well, and we were going home. I saw it as clear as if I were living it. Then, it was over, and my eyes focused on a bouquet of flowers on the altar. They offered another splash of color in the subdued, tranquil room. What did they signify? Well wishes for a child that was sick? —the memory of a child who had passed? No!

What did it all mean? Was it a vision, a dream, or a hallucination? I had never seen a vision before, as far as I knew. I always thought visions were reserved for Christians with a deeper or more charismatic faith than mine.

Why would God talk to you, Kip?
Isn't that why you came to the chapel?
What were you praying for, then?

I both rejoiced and doubted what I saw as rapidly as the sides flip on a spinning coin. Finally, however, I decided that what I saw meant that Chance was going to recover. That had to be it! I clung to that vision of hope as I got up and returned to be with Marti and Chance. I kept the vision to myself, though, as a secret guarded closely to the heart. Just in case…

I'M more of an emotional man, and I often take a prayerful approach to many problems. Marti, on the other hand, preferred to take a more scientific approach. While I was in the chapel on my prayer vigil, Marti requested all the information she could find from the hospital library about HUS and E. coli O157. She planned to attack the problem by arming herself with as much knowledge as possible. Whose approach was better? It didn't matter; we were a team, and we complemented each other well.

When I returned from the chapel, however, Marti was back in bed with Chance holding him in a position she would maintain without respite until the following morning.

Chance's urine output was decreasing already—an ominous sign. Were Dr. Stanga's fears coming true? The nurses gave Chance a dose of Lasix in his IV in the hopes it would stimulate kidney output and reduce the stickiness of his platelets. This had the unfortunate consequence of ramping up the intensity of his abdominal problems. Much of Chance's care went like this: solve one problem and cause another. It was a cruel puzzle that apparently had no solution.

The Lasix medication caused his cramps and diarrhea to come every five minutes; it was incredible to behold. My son only weighed around twenty-three pounds when the ordeal started. How much of his essence could he afford to lose like this?

At seven o'clock that evening, a nurse inserted a catheter into Chance so that his urine flow could be monitored. We then dimmed the lights, hoping that would calm him down and help him get some sleep. With Marti in the bed and me in a nearby chair, we settled in for what we anticipated to be another long night.

I have no idea how I was functioning by then; it must have been adrenaline only. When would I be able to sleep again? I didn't know. Did it matter? No.

I sat in the chair and tried not to become fixated on the stream of urine flowing down Chance's catheter tube, but I couldn't help it. My mind was full of wild images: South Dakota, the breakfast, flowers on the altar, exploding asteroids, drops of urine, and my premonition in the chapel.

Hold on to your vision, Kip, I told myself. *You are going to carry him out of this hospital.*

CHAPTER 6

Molly

AS much as I tried, I could not avert my gaze. I couldn't stop staring at Chance's flow of urine through his catheter tube the second night at The Children's Hospital. Ever since Dr. Stanga told us the next forty-eight hours were crucial to determining whether Chance would lose the use of his kidneys, I was obsessed. The kidney watch had begun.

Marti slept in Chance's bed with him, and I sat as quietly as I could in my chair. Despite my own lack of rest, I insisted that Marti close her eyes and try to sleep. Chance needed her calming influence, and I promised I would wake her if anything happened.

A relative peace and calm overcame the room after we dimmed the lights. The heart monitor glowed quietly as it kept its silent vigil along with us. I felt anything but calm on the inside, though. Numerous thoughts fought for attention in my mind while I stared at the drops of urine in the collection tube.

Drip...drip...drip...drip...

What if Chance spent years on a waiting list because he needed a kidney transplant? Would he ever be able to play soccer or baseball? What would years of being hooked up to dialysis be like for him? My mind was starting to feel warped. My body had an irresistible urge to fall asleep, but my mind would not let it—too many thoughts, questions, and fears. My emotions were too raw for me to find rest.

Drip...drip...drip...

My over-active mind returned once more to the recent South Dakota trip. What could have happened? Bear Country...Mount Rushmore—a week ago to the day we experienced that fantastic family time in the Black Hills—breakfast, vow renewals, and time spent with friends.

Drip...drip...

Breakfast...breakfast the morning we went to Mount Rushmore, Chance and I shared a skillet-style dish together. It had ground beef in it. Everyone else had pancakes. Crash!

Drip...

A car accident had interrupted our breakfast that morning. Before we were served our food, an automobile accident took place just outside the restaurant. The unfortunate driver tried to drive his car up a telephone pole and had to be cut out of the vehicle by emergency workers. Everyone in the restaurant went out to gawk, including the wait and kitchen staff. The crash...

No more drops. Was that all?

Drops began flowing down my face, instead of Chance's catheter tube. Tears came when the helplessness of my situation overwhelmed me. Was that it? Did I just witness the failure of my son's kidneys? The time was about nine o'clock in the evening.

Do something!

I sat there frozen in my chair for quite some time, willing another drop to fall down my son's catheter tube by staring at it with unblinking eyes. I could not force my muscles to move or my mouth to open.

Take action this time! Don't wait too long again!

Gnawing thoughts of helplessness tormented me as I sat there. I felt like a captive in a nightmare, willed into inactivity by an evil, outside force. I knew I had to tell somebody, a nurse, Marti, anybody, but I still couldn't move. I could not overcome my denial; I insanely felt that if I just sat there long enough, the hoped-for yellow drops would miraculously resume falling down the tube.

Get up! Tell somebody...tell someone your son's kidneys just failed.

After about a half an hour of despair, hearing every second of the clock tick away in my head, I woke Marti up around nine thirty to share the news with her. She argued with me vehemently, claiming that urine really was flowing. I tried to explain that the drops she saw were just condensation on the sides of the tube. Denial had definitely set in for Marti, and I could not convince her. I couldn't blame her, though, considering the thirty minutes of misery I just spent in the chair. She told me to wait and see, but nothing changed in the tubing as the minutes passed.

Crash! Things went haywire, and we learned just how important a person's kidneys are. Alarms went off in Chance's room all over the place. His heart monitor went crazy, as his heart rate skyrocketed above two hundred beats per minute. That blasted thing kept going off. Nurses were in and out all night taking blood, turning off the alarms, or adding medicine to Chance's IV. Low sodium presented the most serious issue of the night. Sodium, an important electrolyte found in the bloodstream, drops in concentration when the kidneys fail and fluids build up in the body.

It was a crazy night. Once again Marti and I went without sleep. That night, though, we met a very special nurse named Molly. She came on duty right before Chance went downhill, and we felt lucky she was assigned to us. Molly supported us immensely with her calm reassurance. She had an innate knack for silencing the panic buttons in our heads as much as she silenced Chance's heart monitor alarms throughout the long night.

We grew to love Molly; her compassion was crucial to us on several occasions during our stay.

INSTEAD of our expected visit from Dr. Stanga the morning of Saturday, August 6, we received a visit from a team of The Children's Hospital surgeons. All of them, I think. They informed us that they needed to surgically insert some tubes into Chance's stomach for peritoneal dialysis. Their plan included surgery at three o'clock later that day, waiting a day for the incisions to heal, and then beginning dialysis on Sunday.

That was hard news to hear first thing in the morning, and the day-long wait until surgery time was unbearable. I wish they could have just taken him for surgery right away that morning instead of making us wait. It was very hard. My concern at the time was that any delay in beginning dialysis would have serious consequences; I was very nervous. We passed the day waiting with little change in Chance's condition. He continued to be extremely lethargic with hourly bouts of diarrhea.

Finally, the surgery team came to get Chance at three o'clock that afternoon. Marti and I held each other and cried when they left. The parting was tough on Marti who had been holding him close and feeling his heartbeat for over two days. I was inconsolable in the surgery waiting room. I tried to watch football on TV but that didn't help, so I just paced and paced. Marti sent me back to Chance's room with orders to go to sleep. I think she was starting to worry about my well-being.

On the way back to Chance's room, I took notice of my surroundings at The Children's Hospital for the first time. There were red wagons everywhere with children in them being pulled by their parents. Almost all the wagons had IV poles attached to them. It was difficult to see; each red wagon represented the story of a child who was sick and in pain.

Seeing the parade of red wagons inspired me to visit the chapel again. I sat in the same spot as the day before; I noticed the flowers on the altar were different. I prayed for about twenty minutes sitting in silence, asking God to give Chance the strength to endure surgery and the doctors the skill to perform it.

I finally returned to Chance's room and waited there for Marti to call when surgery was over. Not long after I arrived her call came—so much for getting some sleep.

CHANCE'S mood after surgery surprised everybody, even Dr. Fitzgerald, Dr. Stanga's resident physician. He seemed as alert and responsive as he had ever been since checking into the hospital, even to the point of sitting up between Marti's legs in bed and sucking on a Popsicle. Dr. Fitzgerald explained to us that the surgery to place the dialysis tubes went well, and she offered us her hopes for a quiet night.

Despite his improved mood, Chance's physical appearance didn't inspire as much confidence. He was starting to retain fluid due to his lack of kidney function. His cheeks looked uncomfortably bloated and puffy. I entertained an alarming thought about that girl in the original Willy Wonka movie that poofed up and floated away. I sincerely hoped it wouldn't come to that! Whoa…sleep deprivation…

We finally felt like we had reached a calm situation and relaxed enough to turn on the television in Chance's room. But, our respite was short lived. Around eight o'clock Marti noticed that Chance's breathing was becoming shallower, and his heart rate was increasing. She called the nurse in to check him out. The nurse downplayed the condition and tried to reassure us by saying Chance was just still recovering from surgery.

That didn't satisfy Marti at all. She looked at me and told me to find Dr. Fitzgerald. I didn't want to undermine that nurse's authority, but sometimes parents need to trust their instincts and be their own advocates. I trusted Marti's assessment of Chance's condition more than anybody else's. I agreed to look for Dr. Fitzgerald.

I walked down the quiet hallway, slipped past the nurse's station, and found the doctor conversing in the break room with another staff member. I hovered outside the door, feeling foolish and indecisive. Marti seemed to have lost trust in the nurse assigned to us that evening, but disturbing Dr. Fitzgerald didn't feel quite right, either. I waited outside the break room door hoping the doctor would leave and I could speak with her. Frustrated, I gave up and returned to Chance's room, just to make sure…

Marti had a panicked look on her face when I arrived. I felt my heart and stomach trade places within me. Her grave concern convinced me that I made the wrong choice to return without Dr. Fitzgerald, so I turned to leave once more. As I did, I heard a scream.

Marti was screaming. I turned and saw Chance's face turning blue. Marti screamed, "He's not breathing!" Without hesitation I ran from the room at top speed, motivated by fear and adrenaline.

My son is not breathing…run! My wife…run! Hallway…nurse's station…break room…bang on the door.

Dr. Fitzgerald, he's not breathing!

What? He was great half an hour ago…?

He's not now! Run!

The doctor and I ran back to the room together. Already, personnel from all over the hospital descended on Chance's room: the head nurse, X-ray techs, PICU nurses, doctors, and staff from all over. I never got back in the room—I was trapped outside.

I was frantically worried about Marti in there by herself with all these other people. She was still holding Chance, as far as I knew. I had no idea what to do. I stood outside the door listening, trying to make sense of all the commotion I heard. Where was Marti?

Then I saw our new favorite nurse, Molly, turn the corner in the hallway, heading for the nurse's station. She was just starting her shift. She carried a Taco Bell bag in her hands.

I ran toward her screaming, "Molly! Molly you have to get in there! You have to get Marti!" She had no idea what was going on but sensed the urgency of my actions. I blurted out, "Chance…not breathing…get Marti!" Molly nodded and acted immediately; she dropped her Taco Bell dinner on the hall floor and ran into the room.

What was happening in there?

Seconds later Marti emerged looking as pale, scared, and fragile as I've ever seen her. Her legs barely functioned, and her knees buckled as I caught her. We propped each other up and stumbled to a nearby waiting room. Marti could barely walk on her weak knees; I almost had to carry her there.

Marti was near hysteria. Between ragged, shallow breaths she cried, "He's not breathing…he's not breathing!" The wild, panicked look in her eyes matched my own fears, but I knew instinctively in that moment that my wife needed me to be strong. For a terror-filled five minutes, I looked into my wife's pleading eyes and wracked my brain for something I could do or say to help her through this worst of all moments.

Don't let your wife down, like you let your son down! She needs you; do something!

I didn't have the strength, but I had the will; I would have done anything for my wife to bolster her crashing emotions. And then, the spirit led me to an idea. I had it! I held her head by her cheeks in my hands and pulled her close. We touched noses as I looked her in the eyes and told her what we were going to do when Chance came home from the hospital.

We are going to throw such a big party....

PLANNING, crying, waiting, dying, clinging, pacing...anguish. We clung to each other there, waiting frantically for news in what must have been the longest forty-five minutes of our lives. During the crisis, a doctor whom I did not know hovered in Chance's doorway. He stuck his head out once, and I pounced on him for an update. "They're still working on him," was all he would say before he returned his attention to the room.

Still "working" on him? Oh, God!

Still working...

Working...

We stood bolt upright when the head nurse emerged. I tried to read her face but could not. I have never been so scared. Our hearts and breath stopped in our chests, and I thought the nurse would take forever to walk the distance between us. Marti and I could barely stand. We propped each other up and braced ourselves against the bad news we felt was sure to come.

"He's breathing comfortably now," she said.

What?

We exhaled, blinked, and stared at her. We could barely hear her words due to our heartbeats pounding inside our eardrums. She invited us to return to the room to see our son.

When we did, what I saw made me break completely down. I cried uncontrollably at what I saw.

Molly!

She was holding him in much the same way Marti had been doing the entire time we had been in the hospital. The heroic nurse knew what Chance needed most: the comforting touch of a mother, and she acted as Marti's surrogate during his moment of crisis. I may never be able to fully comprehend the compassion she displayed for our son in that moment. I couldn't stop crying.

Molly stood up, silently handed our son back to Marti, and left the room. She wasn't even officially on duty yet.

CHAPTER 7

A Shot in the Arm

THE next few hours were a blur. Dr. Fitzgerald, as a precaution, ordered Chance transferred to the pediatric intensive care unit. We spent the time hearing explanations of what happened, making preparations for the move, and taking deep, deep breaths. Our heads felt like they had been turned inside out.

Marti and I desperately needed a break. We were exhausted from the endless parade of emergencies Chance's illness and hospital stay threw at us. But, it was not to be. Immediately after Chance resumed normal breathing, thanks to Dr. Fitzgerald, we began the laborious process of transferring him to PICU. But first, we received the explanation for why he stopped breathing normally:

His throat was swollen from the surgery to insert the dialysis tubes; the morphine he was given for his pain was not being metabolized by his inactive kidneys; and fluids had built up in his tissues. These three conditions caused a potentially deadly constellation of problems. Dr. Fitzgerald and her team saved Chance by intubating him, administering steroids to reduce his swelling, and hand pumping his stomach.

Marti and I marveled at the miraculous appearance of all those people who worked together to save our son that night. I'm not sure how they knew to show up when they did. Neither Marti nor I remember hearing an overhead page, or anything like that.

Maybe it had something to do with me running down the hallway screaming like a lunatic? They must have a crazy-father alarm button behind the nurse's station desk.

Marti and I expressed our extreme gratitude for everyone's heroic efforts. At the same time, however, we also felt obligated to share our concerns regarding the other nurse who had downplayed our concerns about Chance's sudden deterioration. We asked that the nurse not be assigned to us again. What about Molly, we asked? Could she be assigned to us whenever she was on duty? We felt much better after the supervisor assured us that she would make it so.

We had nothing against that other nurse; we just wanted the best care possible. We felt the head nurse's openness to our request spoke well to the quality of customer service and care provided by The Children's Hospital.

We loved Molly, especially after the episode we just endured. She had the same motherly concern for Chance that Marti did. He needed that. A mother's love: there's nothing like it; it's irreplaceable.

I will never be able to thank Molly enough for what she did for us.

THE preparations for transferring Chance to PICU took over three hours. Once there, Chance was placed in a crib. That meant that Marti could no longer share a bed with him. The separation was very hard on both of them. A ridiculous number of tubes, cords, bells, and whistles were hooked up to our son. He looked so pathetic. Just a few short weeks ago, he passed his eighteen-month checkup with flying colors, and now his survival seemed very uncertain to me.

Marti and I were near the breaking point. We both felt crushed by the emotional and physical toll that jumping from one crisis to another exacted from us. To calm us down, the PICU personnel led us like dazed sheep to their waiting room. They called it the "quiet room" for families. It offered us a chance to be alone, to rest, or to cry.

Our brief rest was over by two o'clock in the morning due to another setback. Chance's electrolytes were critically out of balance. What next? *Oh, God, what next?* The time to begin dialysis had suddenly and ominously arrived. The problem was that the head dialysis nurse was not on site in the middle of the night and had to be paged. *Hurry!*

Marti began crying uncontrollably. She begged the PICU staff to keep her son alive until the dialysis technician arrived. My emotions weren't far behind. We needed good news or hope but had no idea where to find them.

It was too much to bear. The adrenaline had worn off but another crisis was looming, and hope was beginning to fade. Marti and I retreated once again to the quiet area, the windowless PICU waiting room with the 1970s furniture.

It was in that moment that the nameless PICU nurse offered up her bold prediction. Just as Molly knew what Chance needed; this nurse knew what we needed: a large dose of confidence shot straight into the arm—the best medicine possible for despairing parents.

"We do *not* let kids die at The Children's Hospital…."

CHAPTER 8

The Big Party

MARTI'S relentless love and support for Chance played a huge role in his recovery, I have no doubt. She joined our son in his bed the instant he moved into his hospital room and barely left his side for four weeks. Her incredible stamina in the face of sleeplessness, intense worry, and the cruel suffering of one spirit-crushing crisis after another will be legendary in my heart forever. This story is as much a tribute to my wife, Marti, as it is to Chance.

How did she do it?

I don't know. The only thing I can think of is that she is a mother. When their children are endangered, mothers enter an emotional place that men will never understand. Perhaps women don't understand it, either. It's instinct. A mother's place is by her sick child's side, never to leave at all costs. Marti entered that place without question or complaint and became our son's precious lifeline.

Chance only responded to Marti the entire time. She was the only one who could begin to calm him and keep him comforted with her soothing presence. In spite of his ear-splitting screams of fear and miserable whimpers of pain that must have broken her heart a thousand times over, she stayed. In spite of the unceasing monotony of changing diaper after bloody diaper, she stayed. She stayed even though she was an important team member at her employer's office and had to take an emergency leave of absence. She stayed even though she had other children at home. She was Chance's mother.

I tried to get her to rest, to eat...to take care of herself...but her single-minded purpose could not be derailed. I couldn't begin to comprehend it, so I just let her be.

I could not have handled Chance's illness without her. Chance was not responding to me; he needed his mother. I could not have comforted him as well as she did. I would not have had the fortitude to change his bloody diapers time after time after time. I was ill myself and collapsed twice from fatigue and physical weakness. Both Chance and I needed her. Seeing her strength inspired me to find mine.

It will be a long time before I can forgive myself for being slow to act in the early days of Chance's illness. Marti, God bless her, has never accused me of this—no blame, no second guessing. We are a team.

Where do people find their hidden reserves of strength in times of crisis? By day two in the hospital, I didn't have any reserves left. By the time Chance stopped breathing on the first Saturday I had missed nearly four nights of sleep. I had also gone days without eating properly because of my intestinal problems. I had nothing left in the tank. Marti was utterly strong and able to keep her emotions in check. I, on the other hand, was a train wreck in progress. I needed Marti's strength as much as Chance did.

Our roles reversed in an instant, however. When Marti stumbled out of Chance's room the night Molly took him out of her arms, I could tell with a glance that she was suddenly at the end of her stamina. It was then that I took over. I don't know where I found my hidden reserve, but I'm humbly thankful I found it. This began a pattern that continued throughout the remaining ordeal. One of us always had the strength to support the other; it worked both ways.

During our longest forty-five minutes, while the hospital staff worked on restoring Chance's breathing, I told Marti we were going to plan a party—the biggest welcome-home party ever. I held her cheeks in my hands and pulled her close. We sat there nose-to-nose and planned our son's welcome-home party. Where did that crazy idea come from? I don't know. Fortitude and strength come from unexpected places. Innovative ways to cope with extreme stress are gifts from the spirit.

In one of the most frantic, stressful moments to that point of our son's illness, I was able to provide the support Marti needed, when she needed it. I am so thankful; she deserved more.

Chance's illness taught me something about my love for Marti. I'm convinced there comes a time in a man's life when his love for his wife may suddenly reach new and dizzying heights. She may do something so utterly endearing that he knows for sure, whether he knew it before or not, that the woman at his side is his soul mate forever. I experienced that moment with Marti *every single day* of our ordeal with Chance.

She held him close to her heart for a solid month and sacrificed her own well-being to do it. Seeing her son in so much pain for so long must have eaten away at her soul much as the toxins ate away at his body, but still she held on. She held on so tight that she didn't want to let go the night his face turned blue and he stopped breathing. The hospital team had to tear him out of her fierce grasp to bring him back to life.

He came back. To be with his Mommy, I'm sure.

Marti, our children need you.

I need you, too.

CHAPTER 9

Leaving Home

I FELT paralyzed, laying there. My limbs were stuck against the cold, hard floor; they were so heavy. Swirls of color and muffled sounds surrounded me. Spinning, floating…stuck—so heavy. A face above me took shape…shadows…movement.

You okay?

No, I'm not. I'm stuck in a nightmare, and I can't escape.

I heard more sounds and saw movement above me.

Sir? Sir?

"Sir, are you okay? Sir? What happened?"

I narrowed my eyes and attempted to focus. There definitely was someone above me asking me what happened. I felt the cold floor tiles on my back. Why was I on the floor?

"I must have fainted," I said out loud. *I like it down here, I think I'll stay…so tired.*

"Sir! What's your name? Do you know where you are?"

Yes, I'm stuck in a nightmare, and I can't wake up.

A burly man wearing green scrubs and a stethoscope around his neck picked me up off the hallway floor outside the cafeteria and held me upright; then, he led me by the arm to the wall and supported me there. He asked me again what happened. I fainted—how embarrassing.

I told him some of my story and mentioned that my son was in PICU and just started dialysis, and that I had been awake for seventy-six straight hours.

My Good Samaritan raised his eyebrows and looked at me funny. I couldn't tell what surprised him more: the number, or the fact that I knew what it was. I had been keeping track, actually. Diarrhea, lack of sleep, and little food intake left me in a near delusional state, probably as raw and unhinged as I had ever felt. Seventy-six hours.

I fainted on the way to the hospital cafeteria seeking food for Marti and me. After the man set me upright, he gave me a stern warning about getting some rest, or soon I was going to be a patient in the hospital.

What hospital? This is Children's, you can't admit me here! But I do know a good room on the fourth floor....

I needed some sleep.

I SAT still for a while in the cafeteria, gathering my thoughts and clearing the fog after hitting the floor. I reflected on the irony that I should faint at that moment. Marti and I had just finished a conversation in which we discussed the necessity of me leaving to manage our lives outside the hospital—and getting some rest. Marti was able to steal catnaps from time to time, but I had been awake for the duration.

We had our three other children to take care of. Shannon and TJ were traveling with their mother in Hawaii that week, and Loryn was staying with her father. Loryn was scheduled to return to stay with us the coming week, however. We also had two dogs that our neighbors had been watching. As we grew to accept the fact that we were settling in for an interminable stay at The Children's Hospital, it became clear to us that someone had to maintain watch over the Moore household.

That person had to be me. Marti was the only person who gave Chance a measure of comfort, so there was no other choice. Plus, Marti wouldn't have it any other way. We were relieved that she was able to request emergency family leave from her employer. I worked as an independent investment advisor, so my schedule was much more flexible.

Even with this decision made, we knew we could use more help in that extremely difficult time. We agreed to send an S.O.S. to Kansas, where my parents lived. When I called, I discovered that they were already three hours down the road. They had made the decision to come long before we asked. Grandparents are great in a crisis, like the cavalry charging to the rescue.

I returned to the pediatric intensive care unit from the cafeteria to check on Marti and Chance. I winced when I looked in on my son; I just could not get used to seeing so many machines hooked up to that little boy. He still looked comatose.

Silvia, the lead dialysis nurse, had arrived around three thirty that morning, Sunday, August 7, after being paged. She immediately got to work setting up the dialysis machine and performing Chance's first procedure. The dialysis process fascinated me; the swishing sounds of the fluids rushing in and out of my son's body were mesmerizing. I tried to engage Silvia in conversation to ask how dialysis worked, but I was too tired and self-absorbed to really understand it at the time.

Silvia performed a type of dialysis on Chance called *peritoneal dialysis.* Utilizing the two tubes that surgeons inserted the previous day, she flushed a special glucose fluid into and out of his abdominal cavity. A membrane sack called the peritoneum surrounds this cavity and holds the intestines and major organs of the lower abdomen in place. Many small blood vessels infuse the membrane; so the peritoneum itself can act as an improvised dialysis filter. Water, salts, and metabolic wastes diffuse out of the blood vessels into the dialysis fluid due to osmosis, the passage of items in solution across a concentration gradient. The used fluid, or dialysate, is removed after a period of time, and the cycle starts over again.

Silvia planned for Chance's first session to last eighteen hours. That seemed like a long time to me, but she said it was required to return balance to Chance's metabolism. It was hard to stay awake while watching the tedious process, so I walked laps around the PICU floor. There must have been over twenty critically ill children in the unit that weekend in addition to Chance. It was hard to see, and I wondered what all their stories were. My family had certainly been through a lot in the last twenty-four hours: surgery to insert the dialysis tubes, Chance's rapid deterioration that led to his cessation of breathing, his transfer to PICU, and now...the dialysis—incredible!

At around seven o'clock that morning I woke Marti up to fill her in on what happened during the first few hours of dialysis. That's when we had our discussion about taking care of our lives outside the hospital. Soon after we arrived at the decision that I should go home each night, I left for the cafeteria in search of food and fainted on the way.

I should have taken a pillow with me.

CHANCE received visitors on Sunday, his first full day in PICU. His older sister, Loryn, wanted to visit her baby brother. The idea tormented us, but we morbidly asked ourselves whether this would be the last time Loryn would see her brother. Marti and I reluctantly allowed it, a decision we were quick to regret. Loryn just stared at Chance with a wide-eyed fear; she did not recognize her pale, lethargic brother with all the tubes and machinery connected to him. Marti tried to explain how all those items were good; they were keeping Chance alive. But it was too much for Loryn to bear, and she left the room crying. We felt very guilty about what happened and decided that would be the one and only visit from any of Chance's siblings during the remainder of his stay in PICU.

We had better luck with my parents, though. We learned our lesson with Loryn and prepared them in advance for what they were going to see. Al and Connie Moore arrived around five o'clock Sunday evening, and we met them in the hospital lobby. We coached them on Chance's appearance and condition as we gowned up before entering the room.

Much as I expected, Al, my father, maintained his composure. He typically stays calm in a crisis and waits until after the fact to display his emotions. He plied me with questions during the visit, wanting to know what the prognosis was and what course of action we were taking. Like me, my mother is more emotional in the moment. She cried softly and whispered into Chance's ear that she loved him. It was hard to watch, but I thought they both handled the situation well.

The time came for me to leave and go home, according to plan. The thought of leaving Chance killed me, however, and I tried to explain that I probably wasn't going to be able to sleep at home either. Marti, my parents, and the doctors would have none of my excuses and sent me home in spite of my complaints. Around seven thirty I left, but not before stopping by the hospital chapel for the third day in a row. That was becoming my secret ritual, my prayer time in the chapel.

I don't know why I kept my daily trips to the chapel a secret. It's one of those mysterious things that people do even if they can't explain why. My prayer time became my sanctuary in the midst of chaos, and I would not go without it.

The beautiful Colorado night welcomed me when I left the hospital for the first time in three days. I felt rejuvenated by the fresh evening air, but it took much willpower to force my steps to walk away from the hospital. I definitely felt as if something was missing: my beloved wife and child. There should have been three people in my car that night, instead of one. The further away I drove, the bigger the hollow feeling in my chest became. I almost turned the car around several times and returned to the hospital in spite of everybody's orders to the contrary. I was returning to my neighborhood and my house, but I was leaving my home at The Children's Hospital.

Good neighbors are like family. They'll do anything for you in an emergency. When I pulled up to my driveway that night, many of my neighbors stood outside waiting for me to hear what news I had of Chance. They gathered around me in the driveway as I told our story; I could not help but break down from time to time from the deep emotions I felt after three harrowing days in the hospital. I was reminded of the way we all rallied around each other as we prepared to evacuate for the Table Mountain wildfire just a couple of short weeks ago.

I owe my neighbors a debt of gratitude, because they did so much for us that first week, like mowing the lawn, taking care of the dogs, and doing our laundry. Most importantly, they provided a supportive, listening ear.

After catching my friends up on the latest news, I went inside and fixed a sandwich. I felt anchorless; the idea that I was not where I was supposed to be intensified as I walked around the empty house. The invisible tug I felt pulling me back to my wife and son was hard to overcome. I called Marti to fill the void in my heart and to get an update. She reported that Chance was resting as comfortably as could be hoped for, and that his dedicated nurse was keeping an eye on him. She was about to settle in for the night in Chance's room.

With that, we hung up, and I sighed deeply as I got in bed. I had returned to my house, true, but I was definitely not home.

I laid my head down on a pillow for the first time in four days.

CHAPTER 10

Speed Racer

CHANCE loves to go fast: everything is about speed with that boy. I was hoping he would like soccer, but I guess that's not fast enough for him. We race everywhere: race to the car, race from the car, race to get to bed, and race to put our clothes on. Each morning we race to the front door at his daycare. "I turned on my rockets and beat you, Daddy!" No wonder: Daddy's got no rockets.

Let's see in a few years if he's that enthusiastic about the tenth grade.

Chance talks about cars all the time. He has just discovered RC boats, too. He says boating is just like driving, except "a lot wetter." He'll probably grow up to be a racecar driver, like my dad once was. It's in the Moore family genes. His favorite Hot Wheels game is "bangem' up crash them." It makes my heart race to think about it—he's not getting his license until he's thirty-one, at least.

It was Chance's heart that was racing during his stay at The Children's Hospital, however. We all wished we knew what to do to get our son to slow down.

I RETURNED to The Children's Hospital the morning of Monday, August 8, eager to hear how Chance and Marti had fared overnight. Chance's condition was stable, I learned, but overall not much had changed. The silver lining to that news was that he was stable enough to return to a normal room on the fourth floor and the "purple team," as the hospital called it.

Marti reported that Chance had trouble with seizures overnight. She said that Chance would shake and twitch all over his body. The medical team said this could have been because the E. coli infection had spread to other organs in his body, particularly the brain. Fortunately they did not last long, and we did not have to worry about neurological complications after that. Chance also had issues with a very low blood platelet count during the night; the possibility of a platelet transfusion was discussed but not actually carried out.

As we left the PICU, I had a chance to speak briefly with the same nurse that made the audacious, confidence-boosting statement to us when we first arrived in PICU. As always, I pressed for more answers, seeking more assurance. I asked her if transferring back down to the fourth floor meant we were out of the woods. She pressed my hand with a good luck gesture, smiled, and said, "Yes, I told you…." She had a wry look on her face, however, and the look behind her eyes said to me, in an unspoken thought, *Yes, but you have a long way to go.*

Chance's departure from PICU felt like a victory, but it was very short-lived. Each day brought a new and depressing problem. This day, it was the uncontrollable racing of Chance's heart. Tachycardia, the doctors called it. "Tachy" means accelerated; "cardia" means related to the heart.

Chance's heart rate was fast enough during his hospital stay, typically hovering between 146 and 168 beats per minute, but sometimes it would soar above 200. This set the alarm on his monitor off—about every five minutes by my estimation. It was very jarring and nerve-wracking and made getting rest for anybody impossible.

The doctors decided to run some X-rays and an EKG to learn what was causing the problem. Results of these tests indicated sinus tachycardia, the most common form of tachycardia, which can be caused by stress reactions to conditions such as blood loss, fever, or dehydration. This can be a serious condition, because oxygen is not delivered efficiently enough to critical areas of the body, including the heart itself, with such a high rate. Unfortunately, this problem continued to plague Chance and confound his physicians for the remainder of his stay.

This was an instance where Chance's tendency toward speed was not welcomed at all. Our speed racer son's heart beat like a runaway rocket inside his little chest. *Fasten your seatbelts.*

Chance looked sunken and hollow throughout the day. His lethargy increased, probably due to the dialysis, which had started up again. Doctors ordered twelve more hours, with two passes of fluid per hour. Every half hour, when the fluid was exchanged, Chance became fussy and irritable. I could tell it was a very uncomfortable process for him.

I stayed with Marti and Chance until nine o'clock that evening. From then on I would only stay at the hospital during the day and return home at night. Before I left, of course, I made my daily stop in the chapel for some quiet reflection. I was becoming a creature of habit.

TUESDAY, August 9 brought yet another unwelcome surprise: the necessity of an additional surgery for Chance. Since being admitted to the hospital five days prior, he had required blood draws every four hours. Doctors assured us that these tests where necessary to monitor Chance's critical metabolic systems. The tests we were most interested in were the blood urea nitrogen, or BUN, and the serum creatinine. The ratio of these two substances in Chance's serum gave indication of the function of his kidneys. Other crucial tests included the red blood cell and platelet counts and serum electrolytes.

To spare Chance the difficult challenge of finding new places to draw blood on his little body, doctors felt that a PICC line was required. PICC stands for *peripherally inserted central catheter*. The catheter served as a permanent spigot inserted into a vein in Chance's body for blood draws. My mind kept envisioning it like a tap on a beer keg. We were assured by the hospital staff that this was a safe and complication-free procedure. Marti and I still had bad memories of the surgery to insert the dialysis tubes and its aftermath, however. Nothing was routine anymore as far as we were concerned. We weighed the decision to permit this second surgery very carefully.

There was more to consider than just the surgery. Chance had other troublesome conditions that gave us pause about the surgery. His red blood cell count was dropping, causing anemia. He also, on that day, had blood glucose and electrolyte levels that were severely out of balance. We were worried that those things might be intensified after surgery. I felt like my life had turned into an evil Sudoku puzzle with no solution, where nothing added up.

Marti and I needed a closed-door conference, so we stepped into the bathroom of Chance's suite. I voiced my grave concerns about throwing another surgery on top of Chance's other problems. Marti agreed but felt inclined to trust the doctors in this case. Then, she did what Marti does best: she did some research on her computer. We eventually concluded that the benefits of a

PICC line outweighed any risks. After agreeing to the surgery, it was scheduled for later that afternoon.

The decision whether or not to begin transfusions for Chance was even more puzzling. We definitely had a fear that any blood transfusions would cause greater kidney damage than had already been done. I could not get the exploding asteroids analogy that Dr. Stanga gave us out of my mind. On the other hand, how do you counteract the anemia without transfusions? It was a horrible paradox.

Asteroids! I felt like I was stuck in a Star Trek episode. Captain James T. Kirk found himself in an unwinnable situation once, too: the legendary computer simulation called the *Kobayashi Maru.* How did he solve it? He cheated. Unlike Captain Kirk, however, I could not reprogram the computer simulation; this was real life, this was my son.

Ultimately, we could not pull the trigger on the transfusion. With the blessing of our doctors, we decided to wait for one more day.

Around three thirty that afternoon, technicians came to prepare Chance for surgery. When they wheeled him away, Marti and I followed as far as we could. We stood hand in hand as we watched our son disappear through the double doors to the pre-op suite. The butterflies in our stomachs were intense.

I needed to make a trip to the chapel to pray, but at that time I had still not told Marti of my superstitious habits. Making up the excuse of retrieving drinks from the cafeteria, I left her. Once in the chapel I sat in my usual seat and prayed, asking God to give the doctors the knowledge and Chance the strength to get through this surgery. I meditated fiercely on my vision of carrying Chance out of the hospital. Over and over again I prayed to God to grant me this wish. I left and returned to Marti, stopping at the cafeteria first to get us some drinks.

This time, the surgery went surprisingly fast. In a mere thirty minutes, Chance had returned to the recovery room. We then felt glad we had permitted the surgery. Cleaning the area surrounding the PICC line was another source of discomfort to Chance, but at least from then on blood draws were much easier for him.

After barely having time to exhale after the surgery, Silvia informed us it was time for another fourteen-hour dialysis treatment. We groaned because we knew it meant another sleepless night for Chance and Marti. The challenges never ceased.

The following morning, Wednesday, August 10, was our sixth day in the hospital. I arrived in a depressed mood, because I had trouble accepting how much we had been through in just six days. Chance's kidney watch was in its fourth day. I was concerned about that but not overly so, as doctors said it might take up to ten days for them to recover.

My son's appearance when I arrived that morning depressed me even further. The poor child looked extremely white, with sunken, listless eyes. Clearly, anemia and dehydration were taking a severe toll on him. The racing heart problem continued relentlessly, as well, peaking frequently above 200 beats per minute. Once again, cardiologists were summoned to assess the issue. Once again, no cause could be determined other than anemia and fluid imbalances. Once again, no solution was offered.

That morning's blood tests brought bad news. Doctors concluded that Chance's anemia had reached an intolerable point and that a transfusion was then inevitable. Despite the possibility that a transfusion might cause more kidney damage, the balance had finally tipped the other way: delaying a transfusion would be even worse. Was this an unwinnable paradox? I seethed with frustration; I desperately wished for a reset button. Where was Captain Kirk when you needed him?

Around ten in the morning, the first of two AB positive bags of packed red blood cells hung from Chance's IV stand. The process took about four hours. Too weak to even notice, Chance slept through the entire procedure. When the transfusion was complete, Chance looked better, with improved color and energy. The haunting thought that we might have just forever undermined his kidneys' chance for recovery lingered in the back of our minds.

Most of that afternoon, Marti set up a website that would keep our friends and family updated on Chance's condition. The Children's Hospital supported the site for us, and it became a crucial communication tool. Keeping everyone updated with news was exhausting—reliving the events over and over again with others made us feel like we were in our own *Groundhog Day* movie. Our cruel race from one crisis to another also added to the difficulty in keeping others updated.

We posted our favorite recent picture of Chance on the website's main page: he wore a bright orange t-shirt and sported a wide smile on his face. The picture is still one of our favorites of him, and we proudly display it in our bedroom to this day. Emails of support, love, and well-wishes poured in from all over the nation after the website launched. We even received notes from people we didn't know and prayers from church congregations across the United States. The support we received helped sustain us, and we felt very grateful.

Around four that afternoon, Silvia rolled the dialysis machine into Chance's room and told us that doctors had ordered yet another fourteen-hour treatment. *Another one!* I glanced at Marti and thought I saw a haunted look on her exhausted face. I could tell she knew that dialysis meant another sleepless night.

I prepared to leave for the night around ten o'clock. Before I left, I asked Marti if she wanted to be the one to return to the house that night. A hungry, eager look crossed her eyes briefly, and I could tell she was tempted, but the moment passed and she said no. She would not leave Chance, because she knew that he would only respond to her. If we took his anchor away, it would only complicate what was already an awful situation for him. I vowed to do what I could the following day to help Marti get some rest.

I left for the night feeling awestruck at my wife's stamina and unflagging loyalty to our son.

OUR one-week milestone at The Children's Hospital arrived on Thursday, August 11, 2005. We had become a part of their family. I recognized many of the other sick children and their families by sight, as I saw them day after day taking their red wagon rides around the facility. I was also on a first-name basis with many of the nurses. I was starting to wonder if the day would ever come when I would not see those faces and red wagons ever again.

What would today bring? I wondered absently as I walked into the hospital. When faced with an unrelenting string of life-threatening crises, the impact they have on you wears off, and you eventually become numb to their effects. It's like a resistance to adrenaline, or something. *More drama today, I'm sure. Bring it on...whatever....*

This day brought even more issues with Chance's high heart rate. The transfusion the previous day seemed to have no effect on this. Still, the doctors seemed stumped and ordered an echocardiogram. A cardiologist reviewed the results and concluded that nothing was wrong with Chance's heart—so, no solution...*again.*

We were thrilled to witness the return of an old problem that day: diarrhea. Around noon Chance began having heavy diarrhea again, after going since Sunday without it. Doctors explained that there must still be toxins or bacteria in his body. This scared us because we worried that we had taken some backward steps, especially in light of the transfusion the day before. At least, this time, his stools were not bloody—small victory.

Also on this day Chance developed a new problem: a distended stomach. This would become more of an issue later in the week. *Sigh—bring it on.*

But my speed-racer boy's speed racing heart continued to be the most annoying problem, due to the monitor alarm going off constantly. I finally just told the nurses to turn the blasted thing off, so that Marti and Chance could get a little peace.

Yes, we know his heart rate is high. We've known it for three days. We get it...we get it.

I ended our first week at The Children's Hospital with my daily pilgrimage to the chapel. I still told no one I was doing this. I thanked God for getting us this far, but this time asked him to tell me when the nightmare would end.

I left without any answers and made my lonely drive back to our house.

CHAPTER 11

The Unspeakable Question

CHANCE'S kidneys had been nonfunctional for eight days by Friday, August 12. This fact became an increasing source of anxiety for Marti and me. The doctor's words about his kidney function resuming in seven to ten days stayed in the forefront; the calendar mocked us as the days without urinating passed by. My mind started playing games with me by saying, *Last week you weren't sure he was going to live; this week he is stable. It's going to happen...it's got to happen!*

The waiting for Chance to resume urinating was excruciating. Everything about Chance involved waiting: wait for test results, wait for surgery, wait for dialysis, wait for answers; my life in the hospital felt like it was seizing to a halt, much the same way Chance's drops of urine stopped dripping down his catheter tube a week ago. One slow drop of frustration fell after another, crashing down on us with loud reverberations, reminding us cruelly that we had no solutions, no answers, and no end in sight.

When I arrived at The Children's Hospital that morning, I could not tell who looked worse, Chance or Marti. My wife's exhaustion was heart-breaking to see. For four straight nights she had attempted to sleep in a chair, with little success. Marti was going on ten days with little or no sleep. Our room had limited sleeping accommodations for parents. Each night, the interruptions by nurses and technicians came with maddening frequency. I recalled how I had fainted almost a week prior from exhaustion and was worried Marti was nearing that point, herself.

When I arrived and saw how bad she looked, I phrased my typical query about how the night went as delicately as possible. Marti responded by saying that Chance had vomited *eight times* since I last saw him. Great.

Marti went on to explain that nurses finally gave him a dose of Zofran, an anti-nausea medication around three in the morning. This caused a brief flash of friction between us, as I could not understand why she did not call me when it happened. She told me she didn't want to worry me, but I reminded her of our promise to each other to keep each other informed at all times. The two of us worked as an incredible team throughout the ordeal, and this, thankfully, represented the only disagreement we had the entire time.

I could see how vulnerable Marti had become due to stress and exhaustion, so I calmly reminded her that my parents and I were there to help her, that she was not alone in this. I sincerely wanted to do whatever I could for her, for she was my life as much as Chance was. The pace she was keeping was unsustainable for much longer, I thought, so I suggested that we reconsider our plan and allow her equal opportunity to return home at night for rest.

Absolutely not, she said.

I knew my wife well enough to know that was the end of the discussion.

Chance looked his usual horrible self that morning. He had just finished a fourteen-hour dialysis treatment when I arrived and was acting irritable and lethargic. His tachycardia problem continued as well. Each day we took chest X-rays to make sure no further complications arose with his heart.

In the evening, the renal specialists decided on yet another fourteen hours of dialysis treatment. We spent the time idly by watching random things on the television. Time passed so slowly. It was excruciating. After Marti caught a catnap and a shower, I left for the night. Marti had already drifted off to sleep in her chair. I kissed her on the forehead as I left: my soul mate.

The next morning, a Saturday, I brought Marti breakfast and a Starbucks. Each day in the hospital felt the same—the monotony was just as depressing as the crisis itself—so I celebrated the weekend by bringing in special food for her. The day was as calm and uneventful as we could hope for with Chance. The diarrhea continued, though. Doctors attributed the condition to the remaining bacteria in Chance's intestinal system. I was starting to get annoyed that, even two weeks into the illness, his stool cultures remained negative for E. coli O157. When I asked them about this, the doctors simply said it was a strain they hadn't seen before. They didn't sound convinced; neither was I.

Monotony, sameness, waiting, anxiety, and more waiting: all for a bug that Chance supposedly ingested but we mysteriously couldn't identify. At least we were having a semi-quiet day, thank God. And then…

Chance's stomach looked so distended that night he looked like he was pregnant, carrying twins or something. It was painful to look at, and I had to struggle to keep my feelings from turning bitter.

Look at this boy! Why can't we identify this thing? What? Why? Have we just discovered E. coli O158, or something?

Chance's heart rate went off the charts, as high as Colorado's Mount Evans.

What did we do to deserve this? Chance was such a good little boy.

He began to thrash around in pain.

Look at his heart rate! And his kidneys? Another couple of days, and they will be toast.

Chance started crying, and he reached out to us with pleading eyes. The message was clear: *Mommy and Daddy please make it stop!* The look in his eyes cut me deeply. I felt as if I had a sword lodged deep in my gut. One twist of the hilt and I would be finished.

I wish I could, son, I would do anything to make it stop. I don't know what to do. I'm sorry, so very sorry. I'm sorry I did this to you.

Chance screamed. "It hurts. *It hurts!*"

Twist.

Chance cried again and again, pleading with us, begging us to make his pain go away. Marti and I were beside ourselves. What could a parent do? Marti tried her best. She held him, rocked him, and cooed as softly as she could. It was no use.

The weekend medical staff didn't know what to do, either. They were not up to speed on Chance's condition yet. They kept prescribing a pain medication that Marti and I knew would have no effect. Nobody was taking any action—it was too much. I snapped.

I felt a molten anger flow hot within me, and I went looking for that young doctor who didn't know a damn thing about my son's condition. I found him and lit him up.

I know more than you about my son! He hasn't ingested solid food for two weeks; he's got a buildup of bile in his stomach. You've got to drain it. This is what I want: abdominal X-rays and a gas-

tric tube. Maybe you should read his chart? Oh, and page our regular doctor, will you?

The doctor finally agreed to the X-ray. However, it took an hour for the equipment to arrive. He begged and screamed the entire time while thrashing about in Marti's arms.

What causes parents to lose hope for their children? What could possibly happen to make them feel like it wasn't worth fighting for a child's life any longer? How many times can one reach that hopeless point and still recover to fight another day?

Marti had reached that point. Tears flowed in waterfalls down her cheeks as my son thrashed about in her arms. Then, she spoke the unthinkable question, a question a parent should never have to utter. "Kip, should we just let him die?"

My heart went cold and stopped beating. I could not fathom why she would ask such a thing, but I saw the look of mortal fear in my wife's eyes and knew she was serious.

"We are being selfish by making him go through all this pain; we're keeping him alive just for us."

Maybe we should just let him die?

I stood there with trembling legs facing my wife and son. I didn't think I had the strength to rise above such intense misery. For the second time since Chance's stay in the hospital began, I knew fate required me to dig deep within to rescue my wife from utter hopelessness.

We do not let kids die.... We do not let kids die....

No! Marti, let me tell you something....

For the first time I shared with Marti my vision in the chapel from the previous week about how we were going to carry Chance out of the hospital, healthy, well...cured. This was the first time I even mentioned that I was going to the chapel, let alone that I had been praying and seeing visions. For a desperate heartbeat I thought she wasn't going to say anything, but then she asked, "Do you really believe that will happen?"

Sharing my vision with Marti had a wonderful effect on me: I felt my confidence growing. I returned her gaze and said, "I have no doubts. I'm not sure when, but I know we will. We will carry Chance out of this hospital healthy."

Marti calmed visibly despite the fact that Chance continued to wail in her ears. She smiled at me. "Thanks," she said. "I just needed to hear you say that."

The unspeakable question had been asked; but thankfully on this night, it didn't need to be answered. My wife's final words on the subject were the most telling:

"I just needed someone to give me hope."

CHAPTER 12

Water Rules

THANKFULLY, Marti and I never had to ask ourselves that dreaded, unspeakable question about our son again. We never asked if we were fighting too hard for his life—fighting for our sake instead of his. From then on, we knew in our hearts our son had the will to live, and our task to support him was sacred and just.

We had plenty of stressful, anguishing flashpoints to go before our story was complete, however; but once I told Marti my vision of carrying Chance out of the hospital as a healthy boy, the dream was ours to share. It became a living force after that, and we used it to mutually encourage each other during those all-too-frequent moments when we found our optimism flagging. A shared dream holds more potential than a secret one.

Once doctors determined his extreme bloating and abdominal pain came from a buildup of bile in his stomach, they inserted a tube to drain it. The quantity of fluid drained dumbfounded us—no wonder he was in such pain! Chance's discomfort lessened by ten o'clock that night and he began to drift into sleep.

I left to find the doctor I yelled at before and apologized for getting angry. He apologized, too, for not moving fast enough, and all was well between us. Later, after Marti drifted off to sleep, I threw a blanket over her and kissed her forehead. I went to the chapel on my way out for the day and prayed.

That night I prayed for God to not let me down. I told him I believed that he put that thought of Chance going home in my head for a reason, and asked him to make sure it came true.

The most important reason the vision had to come true now, I concluded...*is because I just told it to my wife.*

I ARRIVED the following morning to find Chance a very angry child. He cried and screamed most of the day. For some reason, though, I didn't find his wailings quite so disheartening this time. His tone seemed to have changed. In my mind he was just sick and tired of his situation, tired of being hooked up to so many tubes and machines. He seemed more active that day, too, and I found his lusty anger encouraging.

We learned from doctors that irritability is another symptom of HUS as the toxins clear out of the system. We couldn't help but wonder if his illness was starting to take its course. He began to beg for food and water and that encouraged us, too. Unfortunately, he was not ready for either, doctors said, as they would irritate his bloated stomach even more.

Shortly after Marti and I ate breakfast, the best news of the day arrived. I returned to the room and found a big smile on Marti's face; she simply nodded Chance's way and told me to look. He was sucking his thumb! Marti and I hugged each other and shared a happy moment, the first one we could remember in a long time. Both of us cried to see our beloved son's personality rising above his agony. The tears of joy we experienced in that moment helped to cleanse away our recent heartaches.

However, a child sucking his thumb did not signify a cure, we knew. We still had the ominous specter of his nonfunctioning kidneys stalking us, but the sight of him resuming an old habit was an unabashed joy to us and part of the reason we still can't correct him from sucking his thumb to this day.

Despite these minor signs of improvement, the day was still a difficult one for us. Sunday, August 14, at The Children's Hospital, just like all the previous days, passed with its unique set of challenges, scares, and frustrations. It made a father want to suck his own thumb.

Parents are trained to respond when their child is hungry or thirsty, so we found Chance's calls for food and water hard to resist. Around four in the afternoon Chance received a CT scan to check for intestinal blockages. Technicians found none. Despite that fact his stomach soon became extremely distended again. He began screaming and thrashing in much the same way that had caused our meltdown the previous day.

Once again I felt the heat of helplessness rise within me. We already had a tube in his stomach, so we could not fathom what the problem was this time. Just like the previous day, we ordered X-rays and waited. Seeing your child thrash and scream so much just makes your skin crawl with misery. I thought I might rub the skin raw off my knuckles from so much hand-wringing.

X-rays this time showed the already existing tube had slipped into the small intestine, where it did no good. Once adjusted, the tube slowly reduced Chance's pain as another impressive amount of bile drained away.

Another day, another challenge, another trip to the chapel before I departed. I found my usual seat in the second row and sat alone. I thanked God for the small signs of improvement today and asked him for guidance regarding Chance's kidneys. I closed the ornate double doors behind me as I left and drove home.

THE following morning I drove to The Children's Hospital preoccupied with the calendar. Ten days had passed since Chance last urinated—I convinced myself our time was up. After arriving at eight thirty, I waited until eleven for the renal specialists to examine Chance. I pounced on them with many questions:

> Is there any hope of his kidneys returning?
> What happens if they don't?
> And what would the next step be?
> What percentages of kids don't get their kidney function back?
> Does this mean that we're looking at a transplant?
> Will the Jayhawks win the championship this year?

These questions and more went unanswered on Monday, August 15. Our team of physicians told us to be patient. Hope was not yet lost; ten days was not the point of no return. If we reached twenty-five to thirty days without function returning, then yes. For now, be patient. We'll just take one day at a time and continue with aggressive dialysis they said.

Patience. I was beginning to hate that word. That day it was Marti's turn to prop me up; she told me to stay positive, the best possible outcome could still happen. Her encouragement helped me; we were a team.

This day was relatively calm and uneventful, for the most part. Chance was extremely irritable and clingy with Marti. He kept asking to be held, which was hard with all the hardware sticking out of him. His lethargy returned, unfortunately. Chance's red blood cell count dropped again, and this caused more hand-wringing, as we hoped to avoid another transfusion at all costs.

That night I spent over ten minutes in silent thought after I arrived at the chapel. My mind had made room for my doubts, and I had trouble not dwelling on my misgivings. When I did finally start to pray, I told God that I was sure he was tired of me bugging him and yapping in his ear all the time. However, I warned him that I was going to keep on doing it until my prayers were answered.

DID Chance's diaper have pee in it overnight, or not? That was the question on Marti's mind when I arrived on Tuesday, August 16. The overnight nurse thought so. She placed a bag in his new diaper to catch any urine that might come. A glimmer of hope…maybe? *Patience.*

It was hard to be excited when Chance looked so crappy. He looked very pale and listless. The blood count test that morning confirmed our suspicion that he had become anemic again. His heart rate still had episodes above two hundred beats per minute. The medical team decided to wait another day on the transfusion decision.

Chance continued to beg for food and water. Doctors kept reminding us that neither would be good for him at that point. Denying him those things felt so contrary to our instincts, though. When Marti slipped out for lunch, I couldn't help myself anymore. I gave Chance a few gulps of water. I broke the no-water rule.

I was definitely starting to become a subversive father: dressing down doctors, ordering X-rays left and right; finally, I was now administering a forbidden substance to my son. I convinced myself I couldn't help it; his lips looked dry and chapped, and his eyes looked so sunken. I justified my actions by telling myself that the tube in his stomach would suck it all back up again, anyway. Right?

I waited for the alarms to go off in the hospital and the water police to show up to carry me away, but none came—all was well. More good news: Chance's second prolonged bout with wet, heavy diarrhea stopped that day, and we were all relieved. See? Good karma, no problem.

Talk about good karma—the following day Marti and I would observe our fourth wedding anniversary. I had a sneaky plan, and I confided in the nurse, Molly, to enlist her help. This plan gave me a positive place to channel my subversive tendencies. Excited to put my plan into action the next day, I left for the house after praying in the chapel.

As I drove home that night I contemplated with a wry smile what a pain in the butt I had been at the hospital to that point: running like a crazy man down the halls, fainting in the cafeteria, manipulating the nurse's shift schedules, and now, breaking the no-water rule. The following day, my anniversary, I would break the fire rule.

The Children's Hospital would be glad to get rid of me.

CHAPTER 13

A Red Rose Day

A PROLONGED crisis can tear some married couples apart. Other couples will find the bond between them intensified for the same reason. What's the difference? What equips some husbands and wives to survive a dramatic life episode similar to the one Marti and I did? I don't know, but I am so grateful that we did. Sharing our ordeal with Chance as a team solidified our relationship like no other circumstance could. A weekend marriage retreat in the Rocky Mountains would have been a lot less trouble!

Some couples do not cooperate well in the best of times. Even after weeks of experiencing insane stress while fighting for Chance, we rarely had an unkind word for each other. Our only misstep was our one disagreement about what constituted an update-by-phone-call worthy middle-of-the-night situation the night he vomited numerous times. No small accomplishment when you consider the many other opportunities we had to be impatient or petty with each other during frequent moments of heart-rending stress.

We took advantage of none of those opportunities to lose our respect for each other. When you've gone four days without sleep, and your eyes feel like they're being sucked out the back of your head, how do you keep a civil tongue in your mouth for your spouse? I don't know how, but we did.

I wish I could quantify what makes our partnership work. I hesitate to call it luck, for that would diminish the efforts we both have contributed to our relationship to make sure it does work. Finding the right person in the first place might constitute luck; keeping the right person takes hard work and commitment. Our marriage is the second one for both of us. Perhaps that's the key: neither of us takes love and happiness for granted. Now that we have both of those things, we vigorously defend them.

A wise person once said that if a husband and wife can wallpaper a bathroom together and still be on speaking terms when finished, then their love is a good one. After what Marti and I experienced together the month Chance was sick, I'm guessing we could successfully cover an entire house. Both Marti and I are passionate, strong-willed people. I think that's one of the reasons we are together: we are reflections of each other. Passion runs strong within us.

Passion turned inward is conflict; passion turned sideways is misunderstanding. Marti and I are human; we're not perfect. We've experienced arguments, as all couples do, and we've also had our share of miscommunications. However, we seem to do well in a crisis. Whenever we have an argument, we joke that we should go to the hospital to resolve it. Either way, we typically learn what went wrong as quickly as possible, fix the issue, learn something new, and then move on without resentment.

Passion turned parallel is teamwork; passion turned outward is love. I didn't care how many days we had spent in the hospital with our son, or how tired or ragged we were. I didn't care how discouraged we were about Chance's discomfort or long-term prognosis; we needed to celebrate our fourth anniversary, and I was going to make it happen. We had to turn the passion toward each other, if only for one night. We could only run in parallel for so long before we got sideways. Taking care of ourselves would help us take care of Chance. He needed us.

I ARRIVED at the hospital the morning of August 17, 2005 eager to put my sneaky anniversary plan into action. I felt intensely close to my wife during our month in hell and couldn't wait to give her a celebratory hug and kiss. She made countless sacrifices for Chance's sake during that time, and I have never been so proud of her.

Little did I know, however, that Marti planned on surprising me, too. After arriving that morning, my beloved wife gave me what every man hopes for on his anniversary: a bag of urine… make that a Polaroid picture of a bag of urine. Marti sure knows how to give a good gift.

Yes, Chance had peed in the middle of the night, and we were ecstatic. The hospital staff gathered in the room to observe my reaction and wish us a happy anniversary. My son's surprise urine output represented a huge potential milestone for us, and the joy left me speechless. We danced in each other's arms in celebration while nurses and doctors clapped and cheered around us. Then, I found my voice and peppered Marti with questions:

What does this mean?

How much pee was it?

Is the nightmare over?

How could you keep the secret for so long?

Where did you get the Polaroid camera?

Marti just smiled an endearing grin. She responded by saying that since she wasn't able to go shopping, she figured a bag of pee would be the next best thing. I loved her so much; she did the best she could with what she had to honor our special day—her love was the best gift ever, but the picture proof that my son was getting better came in a close second.

We celebrate the little things, we celebrate the big things, and we never forget the love. We'll always have August of 2005 to remind us that we can endure anything as long as we have each other. I am humbled. She honors me so much by loving me; I pray that I will always measure up.

The renal specialist came by next to share in our good news. He said that once a patient starts urinating again, improvement will often take place in as little as a few days. Our happiness intensified on hearing his words. My sneaky anniversary surprise could not be compared to this, but around five o'clock that afternoon, I put my plan into action anyway.

After telling Marti I needed to leave on an errand, I left the hospital to pick up a nice meal from a local restaurant. I returned with the food and one red rose in a vase and proceeded to set up my romantic dinner on a table in the break room.

I started giving single red roses in 1997 by placing them on my grandparents' gravesites when I marked special moments in my life. I wanted them to know that I celebrated with them, even though I missed them. Moving to Denver from Topeka, Kansas was bittersweet because I could no longer continue the practice. Then, on March 11, 2001, I proposed to Marti on Grandma Rossie's birthday. I told Marti about my red rose tradition on that night and she cried.

I gave Marti her first red rose along with her engagement ring. Besides promising to be her loving husband, I promised her she would be the beneficiary of the red rose tradition from then on. She said yes, and we got married on August 17—Grandma Ginnie's birthday—I'm a sentimental guy, I guess.

Since then, every time something good happens in our lives—and on special occasions—I give Marti a red rose. She received one when we discovered we were expecting Chance. That was a red rose day if I ever saw one, and so was our fourth anniversary. *Celebrate the small things, celebrate the big things...never forget the love.*

The break room down the hall from our room on the fourth floor of The Children's Hospital was wallpapered in blue. It had a couch and a round table in the center with a couple of hard-backed chairs. There was a microwave in the corner, and the room typically smelled like popcorn. This was the same room Marti and I retreated to when Chance stopped breathing eleven days before. We planned his homecoming party in that room. Now, were going to have a party of a different kind—a great place for a candlelight dinner.

I placed a blue tablecloth over the table and set two pillar candles on either side, and then I signed a card for Marti and put it on the table, too. I placed a single rose in a vase in the center. Everything was in order: dinner from Chili's, plastic tableware, and chips 'n salsa—perfect. The little table was quite crowded. The last task was to light the candles, which I did with anticipation. The night of romance I created almost made me forget why we were in the hospital.

Finally, I found Molly at the nurse's station. With her in tow, I returned to Marti in Chance's room. Molly had agreed to stay with Chance while I kidnapped my wife for our party. She had worked the day shift that day but agreed to stay late just for us so we could have our private time together—another example of the compassion Molly displayed to us while we were under her care.

Marti was very pleased by our dinner party. My sneaky plan was executing as expected…so far. We walked hand-in-hand down to the break room. I saw an anxious looking security guard walking toward the break room at the same time but thought nothing of it. We walked up to my prepared table, and I said, "Happy anniversary!"

Marti laughed and her eyes sparkled, and she asked me how I had pulled it off. She looked genuinely pleased and happy that I had done this. I loved hearing her laugh again; the sound of her laughter soothed my soul.

But in nearly that same moment, the security guard pounced on me. "Sir, are these your candles?" I gave Marti a quick, panicked glance. She shrugged. Her dumbfounded look told me I was on my own.

Yes, they are my candles.

"Sir!" he sputtered. "What were you thinking? Do you know how many flammable items there are in a hospital?" He huffed again. "Oxygen! Do you want to blow the place up?"

Without hesitation, I reached down and blew out the candles. I apologized with a very red face for my poor judgment. So much for romance—I was intensely embarrassed.

Sorry! I'm so sorry. I wasn't thinking. Hey…would you take our picture?

Rolling his eyes at us, the guard snapped our picture, but not before he agreed to let me relight the candles for the shot. I think my bold request disarmed him. The picture was horrible, way out of focus, but I didn't have the guts to ask twice. The grumpy man sighed deeply and walked away mumbling "Happy anniversary" under his breath.

Marti and I sat down and enjoyed our un-candlelight dinner and, among other things, shared a good laugh at my expense. Nothing was going to ruin that night for us. That particular anniversary dinner will always have a special place in my heart. We never thought we'd ever be spending an anniversary like this! During our meal we reminisced on our marriage, and we reflected on our decision to have Chance. Marti reminded me of the story about how we decided to have him, because at first I was reluctant to have another child—maybe more than reluctant....

I remembered sitting in the marriage counselor's office armed with mental notes and bullet points for my argument against having a child together. When the counselor said, "go," I launched into an impassioned, rehearsed speech that lasted thirty minutes and left me breathless. I had many good arguments against having another child, and I was confident Marti could not possibly overcome them all. I had thrown Marti a one-hundred-mile-per-hour fastball that she could never hit.

The counselor blinked and turned to Marti. She looked slightly taken aback. "How do you feel about that, Marti?" she asked.

Marti stared straight ahead and calmly said, "Before we got married, he promised me we could have a child together." Not only had she refuted me in less than thirty seconds, she blasted my fastball out of the ballpark. The counselor returned her gaze to me. "Is that true, Kip?" she asked.

We conceived Chance three months later.

Marti asked me that night if I was glad we had Chance, in spite of the adversity we experienced the previous thirteen days. Without hesitation, I said yes. Countless times since then I have been filled with love for Chance and turned to Marti and thanked her for encouraging us to try for another child—the best decision we ever made.

We had a loving, special dinner that night. Instead of dwelling on the sorrow of our situation, we made the time to celebrate in spite of everything. How crucial was that for us? We recharged our spirits which, in turn, bolstered our courage. I was not going to miss the occasion of our anniversary for anything.

Passion turned parallel is teamwork; passion turned outward is love.

I felt much freer in spirit when I went for my daily pilgrimage to the chapel that night. I thanked God for the recent signs of improvement in my son. I also thanked him for giving me Marti. Coping with our son's illness together, solidified our love and respect for each other tenfold. Our teamwork was a gift from God, and I thanked him for that also. I was so happy to have found her and to know that we would always be together.

The load on my heart was much lighter that night after celebrating my anniversary with my beloved wife, an illegal candle, and a photo of a bag of urine. I thought for sure this whole blessed nightmare was truly about to end.

CHAPTER 14

Premonitions, Patience, and Prayer

I'M just an average guy.

I don't feel like an instrument of God. I have done nothing to deserve any special favors from him. I spend as many Sunday mornings on the soccer field as I do in a sanctuary.

I am a man of feeling. Marti would laugh and say that's an understatement. In the early stages of Chance's illness, I was a basket case of emotions, while Marti held to a calmer, more even-minded approach. Sometimes I ask myself if that's why I was more prone to seek help from a higher power. Did that also make me gullible? Why did I think my dream of carrying Chance out of the hospital a healthy boy was foresight instead of wishful thinking?

I am not a patient man. I think a doctor's favorite word is "patience." Wait for this, wait for that, wait and see...wait for my son to die. I am not a doctor, the best I could do to find patience was to implore a higher power to intervene.

I am a man of superstitions. It's funny what people cling to in a crisis. For the longest time I would only walk around the hallways of the fourth floor in a counterclockwise direction. Silly. And every single time I visited the chapel I sat in the same seat: right side, second row, first seat. God doesn't have anything to do with superstitious people, does he? Does he listen to people who sit in the last seat of the fourth row on the left side?

I never had a premonition about a life or death matter before. That's why I found my vision about Chance both heartening and unnerving at the same time. Perhaps that's one of the reasons I kept it a secret for so long. Some people don't take premonitions seriously. The vision I had the first day in the chapel of carrying Chance out of the hospital some day was so important to me, however.

I had a strong feeling that Kansas would win the 2008 national championship. But it was a hunch—it wasn't nearly as vivid as the scene of triumphantly escorting Chance from the hospital. That hope was sorely tested when Kansas trailed the game by eight points with just over two minutes to go. Marti will tell you that my confidence was waning as I sat with my head between my knees. I couldn't stand to watch the actual game—I sat and peaked through my hands at the big scoreboard hanging from the ceiling. I was shocked when that miracle game-tying shot went in to send the game into overtime. Nothing but net. *It's not over 'til it's over.*

The vision I had about Chance was more significant than that. That's one of the reasons I kept going to the chapel, to keep praying to God to make sure my feelings were legitimate. It was like I was peeking through my fingers at the scoreboard once more, waiting to see if God was going to do what I hoped—heal my son.

I am a private guy. I clung to my habits and visions like a security blanket. I wrapped myself in them the same way we wrapped Chance in his blankets we brought from home. I was selfish. I jealously guarded my dreams and sucked every last ounce of hope out of them before I shared them with Marti. I didn't tell her I saw myself carrying Chance out of the hospital until she had accumulated so much despair that she actually asked whether or not we should just let our son die. If only I had told her sooner, she might not have reached bottom.

I am a man of doubts. I am not exactly sure what faith is. Is faith being a perfect Christian—someone so righteous that God jumps each time they pray to him? Or is faith wearing God down by praying the same thing over and over again like I did? I had done nothing to distinguish myself in matters of faith; I kept my beliefs private, where they did no good to anyone else. I wasn't worthy of any special consideration. When it became clear that a kidney transplant might be Chance's only salvation, I prayed for one.

That meant another family would have to suffer. I didn't think that was what God wanted. Why would he choose us over another family? Was there some karmic balance in the universe that had to be maintained? How do you pray for that? I was so conflicted by that paradox that I simply gave up and started praying for a miracle. Whatever! *Just do something, God. You decide what.*

I wanted a miracle, and I looked for it in the chapel. The chapel of The Children's Hospital was my refuge, and I was always there alone. Never in the twenty-two straight days that I went there to pray did I see another soul in the chapel. It was like my own private meditation room. Amid the noisy chaos that my life had become, the chapel was a peaceful, silent oasis. There were no doctors barking orders there, no heart monitor alarms ringing, no dialysis machines, no cries of pain and suffering. It was to me glassy, calm water in the middle of a violent storm.

I was surprised but pleased that I never had any company in the chapel when I went there to pray. The solitude helped me search for my peace of mind; but I know for a fact that somebody was there each day, because the flowers on the altar changed daily. Somebody on the staff at The Children's Hospital worked hard to keep my private little prayer room clean and beautiful. I focused on those flowers and the stained glass window, and I prayed. I prayed for healing; I prayed for the skill of the doctors; I prayed for strength for Marti and me; I prayed for my sick son's courage. Then when I lost all hope, I prayed for a miracle. I begged for one.

I prayed for a miracle even though I thought myself unworthy. I didn't even know what one would look like when I saw it, but I kept praying anyway. Good thing I am a stubborn creature of habit. Maybe bugging God by telling him your wishes repeatedly without knowing what the outcome will be, and continuing to ask even though you aren't convinced you will receive the answer you desire—maybe that is faith. I really am a man of faith.

I'm just an average guy.

CHAPTER 15

S.T.O.P. E. coli

MARTI'S passion for discovering answers to our horrible situation took her to a different place than me. I went to a spiritual place to seek help from a higher power. Marti went to a place of knowledge to understand and cope with what was happening to us. I think both places are equally valid.

Marti spent countless hours during those endless weeks of waiting researching everything she could about E. coli and HUS. I armed myself with prayer, and she armed herself with knowledge. In addition to learning everything she could about the illness Chance had, she also sought to notify the state health departments of South Dakota and Colorado of what happened to us. Her frustration often morphed into righteous anger when none of the agencies seemed inclined to take action without proof.

Chance's stool lab samples never returned a positive E. coli result, even though the clinical picture was obvious to our doctors. However, without a positive stool culture, we couldn't prove it. At one point, Marti screamed into the phone at some poor health official, "Trust us. We've been in the hospital living through hell. He's got E. coli O157!"

We had *our* proof.

A little girl was airlifted to The Children's Hospital while we were there. I spoke to her parents and discovered that they had eaten in a Rapid City restaurant not far from where we ate the same day. The connection seemed obvious to us. Marti and I finally concluded that our illnesses came from some adulterated beef we ingested the Friday morning before our visit to Mount Rushmore.

Contaminated beef coupled with the inattentive cooking staff who wandered outside to gawk at the car crash outside the restaurant had conspired against us, we believe. I ate most of that skillet breakfast and was ill for weeks; I shared it with Chance, and he nearly died. Marti took one bite and was mildly ill for a few days. The other two kids ate pancakes. Thank God! Looking back at our vacation, we can see now that Chance's first symptoms might have been his unusual lack of appetite during our return car trip.

If we had only known.

DURING Marti's intense research, she discovered a nonprofit organization called Safe Tables Our Priority, or S.T.O.P. She contacted officials from this group during our ordeal, and they provided us with information, support, and comfort. We were so impressed with this organization that we volunteered for them later, serving as fundraisers and helping with their website. I also served briefly on their board of directors.

S.T.O.P. was formed as a grass-roots effort by people either affected or outraged by the Jack in the Box E. coli outbreak of 1993. Although tragic, that episode did much to raise public awareness of the dangers of unsafe food. S.T.O.P. is part of a coalition of organizations dedicated to improving the safety of the nation's food supply through education and public advocacy. The Centers for Disease Control estimates that seventy-six million people get sick each year from unsafe food that they eat. Of those, 325,000 are hospitalized and 5,000 die (http://www.cdc.gov/ncidod/eid/vol5no5/mead.htm; accessed May 13, 2009).

One of the coalition's main goals is to promote federal legislation that will improve the national system of creating food safety standards and investigating outbreaks of food-borne illness. Many of the mechanisms currently in place are outdated, and too many agencies are involved to react efficiently to outbreaks.

In April 2009, citizens and families of victims who have died due to food-borne illnesses shared their stories in Washington, DC to encourage the President and legislators to improve our system for maintaining food safety. The Government Accountability Office, in a November 2008 report, listed food safety as one of the thirteen urgent issues facing President Obama and the 111th Congress (http://www.gao.gov/transition_2009/urgent/). President Obama seems inclined to agree, as he made food safety one of his priorities during his first one hundred days in office. In his radio address to the nation on March 14, 2009, he stated his plan to form advisory groups to advise him on improving food safety laws that haven't significantly changed since they were enacted during the Theodore Roosevelt administration (http://www.whitehouse.gov/blog/09/03/14/Food-Safety/). The 111th Congress is debating several bills designed with this end in mind, including the Food Safety Modernization Act of 2009 (H.R. 875).

Children are among the most vulnerable to food-related illnesses such as HUS. I encourage parents to arm themselves with knowledge about food safety, like Marti did, *before* your children get sick. My sincere hope is that nobody should experience the same thing we did with Chance. Contact your lawmakers to add your voice to those calling for new and improved legislation.

I also encourage parents to learn more about E. coli on the Centers for Disease Control website at www.cdc.gov/ecoli. There you can learn about outbreaks, gain additional information about E. coli, and find out how to keep you and your family safe.

On the S.T.O.P. website, there is a gallery of victim's stories and an honor wall. Most of the stories feature children who were Chance's age when they got sick. You will find Chance's story there along with countless others whose lives have been changed forever due to this horrific illness. One of Chance's photos on his page is our most beloved of him, the famous picture of him in his orange shirt sitting on a rock in a field shortly before he became ill. A cuter child you will never see. But all the children whose pictures are displayed are beautiful. None of them deserved to get sick. Please help us to raise our voices and take action against unsafe food.

Help us keep our children safe. It's our sacred responsibility. Stories like Chance's should never have to be told.

CHAPTER 16

Psalm 62

WHEN is progress nothing but a mirage? When is gain just a cruel tease? How much prayer is too much when you beg God day after day for your son to be healed? Does God ever stop listening?

The optimism we carried with us from the evening of our anniversary seven days before extinguished as quickly as the candle I mistakenly lit in the fourth floor break room.

Snuff.

My son's kidneys produced urine for the first time in twelve days, and we jumped for joy. But, it was not enough? *Are you kidding?*

Seven days later, we were still at The Children's Hospital with no end in sight. *Will someone explain this to me, please?*

Doctors said he could not survive without dialysis if his urine output trickled like a stream withering in a summer drought. We needed gushing, like a river overflowing with Colorado mountain snowmelt in spring.

Okay, when will that happen?

We don't know.

Progress was painfully slow for us the week following our fourth wedding anniversary. In addition to watching his meager urine output with increasing angst and frustration, we also monitored abnormalities in his blood panel, including a triglyceride level that went sky-high. The tube in his stomach began to create concerns of infection, so that was pulled. On the good side, his heart rate seemed to stabilize during this time, and his red blood cell count stabilized and even improved.

By August 20, doctors gave us permission to give Chance fluids and solid food. We were allowed to give him yogurt, crackers, applesauce, and Jell-O. Marti and I were very relieved by this, because we had grown weary of denying food to our son. Of course, once we got the green light, he wouldn't take food. Pretzels were about the only item he would eat. "Bepels" he called them. He won't eat pretzels now.

Physical therapy came next. Chance needed help to restore muscle tone due to spending two and a half weeks in bed. Soon after that, we received clearance to take our first red wagon ride. I remember it clearly. I loaded Chance into his wagon, and I gave him a tour of the entire hospital: cafeteria, PICU, chapel, and the outdoor courtyard. We spent thirty minutes in the courtyard. Seeing Chance listen to the birds and allow the sun to warm his cheeks warmed my heart. I couldn't imagine what it must have been like for him to be cooped up for so many days in his crib.

Overall, though, my heart was still cold with frustration. On August 24, I decided to personally call one of the renal doctors, so that I could have a private conversation without alarming Marti. I asked the doctor several point-blank questions. I asked him about the chances of recovering from HUS. I asked him when we would know my boy's kidneys were okay or not. I asked him when we would know a transplant was required and how long before it could happen.

I got nothing. *Never seen this strain of E. coli O157 before. I don't know how long. You never know.*

I began to mentally shut down after that conversation, preparing myself for the worst.

Our morbid calendar watch continued. Every morning at six o'clock, a nurse would come into Chance's room and take a blood draw. Every morning the results were the same: no improvement in kidney function.

On the evening of August 25, I flipped through my Bible at home. I looked up keywords in the topic index, words that represented things I felt short on: strength, patience, hope, and miracles. I found a passage that looked interesting, Psalm 62. The verses gave me comfort:

Find rest, O my soul, in God alone;
my hope comes from him.
He alone is my rock and my salvation;
he is my fortress, I will not be shaken.
My salvation and my honor depend on God;
he is my mighty rock, my refuge.
Trust in him at all times, O people; pour out
your hearts to him, for God is our refuge.

I read these verses over and over again. They gave me comfort, and I eventually fell asleep.

Chance's appearance and mood improved dramatically over this long week of waiting. We recognized his personality once more; it was a joy to see. I tried to focus on him and his appearance, but when I looked into his eyes I only saw nonfunctioning kidneys.

On Friday, August 26, we had a conference in Chance's room around four o'clock in the afternoon with a renal doctor and

Silvia, the dialysis nurse. They gave us news we never wanted to hear. They told us to prepare ourselves for the very real possibility that Chance's kidneys would never return to full strength. Starting the following Monday, Marti and I would be required to begin a dialysis class that would train us on how to administer the procedure to Chance at home. The class would run eight hours a day for thirty days. *A whole month?*

He also said that representatives of the hospital would be visiting us soon to talk about a kidney transplant and instruct us on how to get on the recipients list. He concluded by saying how sorry he was to give us that news. Chance had become quite popular with the doctors over time. When he got his personality back he ooohed and ahhhed each time they listened to his heart. "Ohhhhhhhh," he would say. It was very cute.

The renal doctor paused in the doorway and looked back at Chance. "You have quite a little fighter, there. He has overcome a lot." With that, he turned and left.

Silvia stayed behind. She explained in more depth what we could expect from the dialysis training. We loved Silvia; she was always so upbeat and positive—a character. Silvia was a free spirit and had a knack for making us smile, even in the worst of times. Neither of us smiled or said much to her on that day, though. We just sat numbly and stared quietly at her. No tears—somber, quiet thoughts. *Dialysis training…bring it on….*

When she left, our silence continued. The day we had been dreading had arrived. We knew it might come. Marti finally spoke. In a dull monotone she said, "At least he's alive and stable." All I could do was mumble in reply, "Yep. We should be grateful for that."

When we found our voices, we began discussing the logistics of the puzzle our lives had become. Marti would run out of family emergency leave time soon; we were afraid she could lose her job as a result. I, on the other hand, had my own business to run. How could I take a class every day for a month and keep it afloat? I would have to hire help, which I could not afford. It was a maddening puzzle. We fell silent again.

We spoke few words the rest of the evening. We tried to put on a smile and a brave face. We were very thankful Chance was alive but felt defeated on the inside. Marti's sister Heather was in town helping out that week. After convincing Marti that she should leave the hospital to be with her the following day, I left for the night by way of the chapel.

I shuffled to the chapel with bowed head. My prayer that night was simple: God, please send me a miracle.

Find rest, O my soul, in God alone; my hope comes from him. He alone is my rock and my salvation; he is my fortress, I will not be shaken.

I needed a rock.

CHAPTER 17

Dad's Watch

I STOOD on the edge of the soccer field, hands in my pockets. The field was cold and damp—chilly. My eyes looked at the young children streaking by in their colored uniforms without seeing. My ears listened to the thump of the ball being kicked back and forth without hearing. Parents came up to me to ask about Chance, ask about our family, share their concerns. I had nothing to say. It was too hard—the foreboding was too overwhelming.

I love watching my son TJ's soccer matches. However, on August 27, I stood on the sidelines huddled in my jacket against the cold, feeling miserable. I wasn't loving soccer that day. As much as I enjoy watching TJ play sports, the match passed before my distracted eyes and was over before I knew it. TJ had two assists in a 4–1 victory.

My lack of enthusiasm for TJ made me feel guilty. I could not get thoughts of Chance out of my mind. I felt small and fragile thinking about the possibilities of Chance never having the same opportunities TJ did: soccer, baseball, or football. He wouldn't even be able to play with the neighborhood kids like other children do. I also felt extremely selfish for Marti and me, and that drove the guilt even deeper. What would dialysis do to date nights, movies, or weekend getaways without the kids? How could we afford specialized nursing care? Where on earth would we find a babysitter? The "what if" and "how" questions kept streaking through my mind like a forward on a breakaway goal.

I felt like I had a soccer ball made out of lead in my stomach. I felt prickly and gloomy, much like the weather that Saturday morning. I could not escape my future...Chance's future.

My blue funk continued as I drove to the hospital. Every action felt like agonizing slow-motion autopilot. When I arrived, I forced a smile on my face on seeing Marti. There was some good news that day: after all this time, I had finally convinced Marti to take a break. Her sister Heather arrived in town to visit Chance and help take care of Marti's daughter, Loryn. After much arm twisting, I succeeded in encouraging Marti to leave the hospital and have an enjoyable night at home with her sister and daughter. I was surprised that she agreed. I could not comprehend what it was like for Marti to be confined in the hospital for so long.

Marti left to be with her sister late in the morning. Finally, she was released from her hospital prison. I said a silent prayer that she would allow herself some fun, and I settled in with Chance. A momentary flash of panic washed over me, because I was worried I wouldn't know what to do with myself all day. *What would Marti do?*

Dad's watch had begun.

Around eleven that morning, I had some business with the nurses, so I briefly stepped out of Chance's room. I saw a man approaching me dressed in the black shirt and white collar of a clergy person. He had a pleasant smile on his face as he stuck out his hand and introduced himself as Father Anderson. The kind man asked about Chance, whom he could see through the door that I had left open a crack.

I returned his handshake and greeting. Then I started telling our story. I cut myself short, though, and apologized. Sheepishly, I said that he had probably heard a million sad stories of children in this hospital. He smiled warmly and encouraged me to continue; his gentle nature was quite disarming, so I finished my story.

When I was done explaining Chance's situation, he asked if there was anything he could do for me, like offer a prayer or Bible verse to share. "Funny you should ask," I replied. "I just read Psalm 62 last night and found it very comforting."

Father Anderson looked at me funny. I felt unsettled, like I had said something wrong or quoted the phone book by mistake. It was starting to feel uncomfortable; I just wanted to get on with my dreary day. The man reached into his pockets with wrists covered in yellow Live Strong bracelets. "I had a feeling that I should put these in my pockets this morning. I think one of them was meant for you."

He pulled out three rocks and held them in his hand as he extended his palm toward me. He explained that one of the rocks was from the Grand Tetons, one was from Yellowstone, and the third was from a local Colorado stream. He asked me to pick one.

He alone is my rock and my salvation; he is my fortress, I will not be shaken.

I chose the beautiful black rock found in the Grant Tetons and thanked him. We shook hands again and went our own ways. The man's kind interest in my story was comforting, but I didn't give much thought to the rock. I shrugged and placed it in my pocket.

That was nice, I thought. *Dad's watch is going pretty well so far.*

Several months later, I remembered the kindness of Father Anderson and decided to seek him out in the chaplain's office to thank him in person and talk with him some more. I was told that The Children's Hospital did not have a chaplain named Father Anderson. *What? The man wasn't imaginary; he gave me a rock.*

The rock is real. We still have it.

He is my mighty rock; my refuge.

THE rest of that afternoon passed in relative quiet and boredom. I felt uneasy, and my spirit was disquieted. The realization came to me that afternoon how much I depended on Marti's vigil with Chance to do the things I was accustomed to doing to soothe my desperate soul. Things like walking around the fourth floor and going to the chapel were not available to me this day, because I was alone. I could have left Chance alone briefly to do those things, but that did not feel right, either.

My forced change of habits caused me to feel unlike myself. I spent most of my impatient energy fussing over Chance and trying all means possible to get him to have a "big urine" diaper. I thought maybe if he had one, I could take a Polaroid picture of it and present it to Marti when she returned.

My appreciation for Marti was very keen that day. Passing the long hours in the hospital watching Chance was lonely work, and she had done it by herself every night for three weeks. After a while, I began to feel punchy and mischievous. I kept pushing fluids on Chance, encouraging him to drink. I even went so far as to play an old college fraternity trick on him.

In my college days, my frat brothers and I would play tricks on each other after a hard night of drinking. We'd pick our victim and once he went to sleep put his hand in a warm bowl of water. Without fail the poor guy would pee in his own bed and wake up wet and confused. It worked every time.

I played that joke on several of my friends. I was a legend in my own mind.

C'mon big urine!

The old standby didn't work on Chance, though. Yes, I played the same trick on my son during his afternoon nap to get him to pee. I was desperate. His stubborn kidneys resisted the frat-house prank, and I felt even more discouraged. I sighed deeply several times; I gave up and decided to behave, or else Marti wouldn't let me stay with Chance alone again.

Not that I couldn't be trusted. Marti and I shared parenting duties equitably in raising Chance. I adored taking care of him, with the exception of changing diapers. However, there were a few times....

I took TJ and Chance to a Colorado Rockies baseball game once. I allowed Chance to eat so much candy we had to leave after the second inning, because he had a bellyache. TJ was helpful enough to point out the error of my ways—a little too late!

Then there was the time when Loryn, Chance, and I watched Marti run in the Denver Half-Marathon. As Marti approached our vantage point, we all got excited and leaned forward through the crowd to see her. Chance tripped on someone's foot and face-planted himself on the concrete. I picked him up and tried to look nonchalant as Marti passed; I waved and yelled encouragement to her. The look on Marti's face as she ran by seeing our son's bloody chin was priceless and a little frightening. Chance still sports a chipped tooth to this day.

Another time I slipped on some ice while carrying Chance and dropped him on his head. That was quite alarming, but I took him to the doctor and he was fine.

Chance is a tough kid—good thing.

I SETTLED in for an evening with my tough boy. No more pranks on Dad's watch. After calling Marti to see if she was enjoying herself, I sat and watched Chance drift into sleep. He was very quiet that night and acted very tired. I tried to get him interested in his favorite book, *What Do Toddlers Do?* But he just lay quietly and sucked his thumb.

I flipped idly through the TV channels hoping to find something to take my mind off our situation. The four additional weeks in the hospital for dialysis training loomed large in my psyche; they haunted me and consumed my thoughts.

My soul was full with a heavy sadness, and I felt near tears when I allowed myself to dwell on our endless nightmare. Yes, it was a good thing our boy was a tough one. He was going to need every ounce of his toughness to face what was to come. I prayed that he hadn't already used up all his strength.

Prayer! I realized that this night was the first night a chapel visit would not be possible. I mourned the disruption of my routine even more. So I did the next best thing and prayed where I was in Chance's room. My prayers that night were for a kidney transplant opportunity. I also reflected on how my meditations had evolved from Chance's pure survival at first; to his kidney's survival, next; and now, finally, to asking for a kidney transplant.

Asking God for a kidney for your son is hard, because it means that another family must know grief and tragedy. It was a terrible paradox that made me squirm. After what we had experienced in the previous twenty-two days, I knew I couldn't wish that on any family.

I did my best to focus on the positives. Three weeks ago, on this very night, Chance was a breath or two away from dying. I needed to be grateful, focus on our blessings, and hope for the future.

THE Denver Broncos played a televised preseason game against the Indianapolis Colts that night. I like both teams, so I thought that would distract me. Just like TJ's soccer match, however, I viewed the game without seeing it. I think the Broncos won. I didn't care. I tried to watch *Saturday Night Live* for a while, but that only lasted for about thirty minutes. Nothing was funny.

When it came time for me to go to bed, I tried at first to get comfortable in the chair Marti had been using for three weeks. It was a small, cloth recliner that looked ragged, as if worn out by thousands of parents who had used it to keep an all-night watch. It didn't work for me, and once again I marveled that Marti had endured so much.

Each room at The Children's Hospital had a window seat with a foam pad big enough for me to curl up on. I figured that was my best bet. It also had a privacy curtain I could use to shield myself from Chance's nighttime nurse visitors. I ended up propping myself against the wall in a fetal position with a pillow. I left the curtain open a sliver so that I could look at Chance. He slept in his crib with his blankets, which we brought from home. He looked like he was in jail behind the silver vertical bars of the crib.

I jumped at the sound of a helicopter landing on the helipad near our room. I looked out the window at our bleak, depressing view of the roof and hospital walls looking for the helicopter but couldn't see it. The sounds of the rotors always spooked me when I heard them; each landing meant another family in crisis, another child in danger. After settling back in again, I finally drifted off into a fitful, uncomfortable sleep, hypnotized by the constant whooshing and whizzing sounds of Chance's dialysis machine.

Marti deserved a medal.

Around twelve thirty in the morning, I was disturbed slightly by a nurse extracting blood from Chance's PICC line. She was quiet, efficient, and left the room as soon as she came. I drifted off again.

I awoke once more. It was around two in the morning. A dim light roused me from a shallow sleep. I looked through the slit in the curtain and rubbed my sore neck.

What's that?

Another nurse—a male one this time. The diffuse light in the room intensified. The nurse was standing next to Chance's bed.

Or was he…? I pinched myself to see if I was dreaming.

I was not dreaming. What I saw that night has caused me more self-doubt and denial than anything I have witnessed before or since. I have replayed the scene in my mind's eye hundreds of times trying to discern its meaning. When I first saw it, however, I could only think one thing: *Nobody is going to believe this.*

CHAPTER 18

Two Parties

WHEN the mysterious source of light departed Chance's room, I sat by myself in the dark, not knowing what to do or think. I was confused and awestruck. Alternating waves of hot and cold chills passed through my body. I sat and wondered: *Did I just witness the miracle I had been praying for?* Time passed by slowly in the dark. All I heard was my own heartbeat and the swishing dialysis machine. I must have eventually fallen back asleep.

At six o'clock I awoke, remembering every detail of what had happened in the middle of the night. Embarrassment started to creep into my thoughts. What would Marti think? I knew she would say that I had officially lost my mind on Sunday, August 28. So I vowed not to tell her. However, I hoped that what I saw was real, and that whatever it was would help Chance recover.

A nurse entered the room for Chance's morning blood draw. A short time later, the renal specialist paid us a visit. He said that he didn't want to excite me too much, but Chance's serum creatinine level dropped for the first time since his kidneys failed. Creatinine is a byproduct of metabolism inside muscle tissue, and is filtered out of the blood by the kidneys. This was one of the serum markers we had been following with intense scrutiny during Chance's hospital stay. The doctor seemed perplexed by this result; he, along with the rest of us, had given up hope of that number ever improving again.

I don't want to excite you too much. At least he didn't tell me not to be alarmed. My heart pounded with excitement, and the warm afterglow from the night before continued. I wanted to tell the doctor what I saw, but held my tongue.

Chance's improvement after the mysterious event in his room the night of my watch was both rapid and breathtaking. Marti and I could hardly dare to believe it. I called Marti the morning after to tell her the exciting news of that first lower creatinine result. We were busting with anticipation but decided to tell no one else the news. I hesitated to tell Marti what I saw. In fact, I said nothing. I kept it to myself behind a veil of embarrassment and guarded optimism. People like me didn't receive miracles. I had too many doubts.

When Marti returned to the hospital, she brought Loryn and her sister Heather with her to visit Chance. We both thought we would bust a gut holding back our news, but we did. We had learned to view any news with a skeptic's eye and didn't want to get anyone's hopes up if the lab results were an anomaly.

That night, Marti resumed her typical role as Chance's overnight protector. I returned to the chapel for a prayer session after my one night away. I sat in my normal spot and prayed. As usual, I meditated on my recurring vision of carrying Chance out of the hospital. I also recited my newfound favorite Bible verse, Psalm 62. Finally, I had one last thing to ask God:

Um, about last night…?

THE phone woke me around seven in the morning on Monday. It was Marti. I could barely get "hello" out before she blurted, "His numbers improved again. Can you believe it? He's getting better!" *Can you believe it?*

I could not. I ran out the door in minutes, wanting to hear the news in person.

I arrived at The Children's Hospital just in time to hear the renal team tell Marti the official news: Chance's lab work was trending downward.

We asked the doctors what that meant. They responded by saying that for the first time in weeks they were hopeful that Chance's kidneys might make a comeback. As always, good news came tempered with caution. Chance still wasn't producing enough urine output. Despite that, the team of doctors decided to take Chance off dialysis that evening.

Say what?

No more dialysis. The time had come to see if Chance's system could jump start itself without the crutch of dialysis to lean on.

Marti and I were breathless. Good news is almost as hard to absorb as bad news is sometimes, especially when all you are accustomed to is disaster.

The doctors concluded their assessment by saying that, if the lab tests did not continue to drop, then Chance's kidneys were likely damaged beyond repair, but they asked us to think positively.

Before the team left the room, I asked them one final question: "We had all given up. Why the sudden improvement?"

The doctor I had addressed shrugged. He said, "No reason. Sometimes it just happens."

I felt chills again. *No reason?* I could think of a reason, but I kept silent. I wanted to tell Marti but couldn't divulge my secret.

Marti and I had been through so much with Chance, we still did not dare to believe our nightmare was over. We couldn't bear the thought of enduring any further disappointments, so we tempered our enthusiasm as much as we could. It was impossible! A mere forty-eight hours prior we were preparing for the worst: dialysis training and interminable waiting for a transplant.

We decided to have dinner out that night. Once again, Molly babysat Chance for us in her off-duty hours while Marti and I slipped away. It was the night before my forty-third birthday. We had no appetite due to our excitement but strolled to a Mexican place near the hospital, anyway. We talked, laughed, and reminisced about our ordeal. The walls of pessimism around our hearts started to crumble, and we began to remember what optimism felt like.

We joked that my birthday was going to be a day to remember. I've had some memorable birthdays, mostly thanks to my parents. My dad treated me to my first trip to Las Vegas on my twenty-first birthday. He lost seven hundred dollars on the roulette wheel to teach me a lesson about gambling, but then took me to see a topless dancer show. Thanks, Dad! My mother was kind enough to remind me my life was half over by placing an extremely large "Happy 40th Birthday" banner over their garage in Topeka. Thanks, Mom!

Marti and I had a feeling that my forty-third birthday would blow either one of those away, for good or bad. We walked quietly back to the hospital, hand in hand.

I left Marti and Chance alone in his room, as usual, to go to the chapel. I paused at the doorway and stared at the spot on the floor where the dialysis machine had stood for twenty-two days. I smiled at my wife and son and left.

Sitting down in my time-honored second row seat of the chapel, I sat alone in silence. I did not pray that evening. I was prayed out. I had played all my cards, putting them face up on the table in front of God. It was his play next. After a month of chaos, the silence in the chapel was about the loudest thing I had ever heard. After fifteen minutes of nothingness, I left for home. On the next day, my birthday, I would learn my son's fate.

I AWOKE around four thirty in the morning on Tuesday, August 30, my birthday. I don't think I ever actually fell asleep; my anxiety was in overdrive. The phone rested next to my ear on the pillow in anticipation of Marti's call. Several times I nearly picked it up to call Marti, because I knew she was not sleeping, either, but I decided to leave her alone.

When the clock reached five forty-five, I knew a nurse was in Chance's room drawing blood out of his PICC line.

Six o'clock: I wondered if this was going to be my best or worst birthday, ever.

6:15: Why hadn't Marti called?

6:25: Nothing yet. It had to be bad news, I thought.

My phone rang at 6:27. My whole body throbbed with my heartbeat; I grabbed the phone with sweaty palms. "Please tell me it's good news," I croaked.

"Happy birthday!" Marti said. *Happy* birthday.

Marti's smile appeared before my eyes as if she were in the room with me. I asked her to repeat herself, so I would know exactly what she meant. She told me his labs dropped again; his kidneys were working on their own. After telling Marti how much I loved her, I hung up and prepared to join her at the hospital.

Tears of joy mixed with droplets of water as I took a shower. I could not tell them apart. I had to lean against the wall of the shower stall to prevent myself from collapsing on my trembling legs.

My son had received his life back; his second chance had begun.

Happy birthday to us.

NURSES and doctors spilled out of Chance's hospital room when I arrived that morning. The celebration had already begun. I felt like a conquering hero as I joined the throng.

Everybody was hugging everybody else. Cheers of "happy birthday" and "congratulations" were on everybody's lips. I had never had such an intense feeling of joy. After hugging and kissing Marti, I said hi to Chance. He wore a blue shirt with stick fish pictures on it. I picked him up and spoke to him, telling him how proud I was of him. I rested the bridge of my nose on the crown of his head and cried. He felt so comfortable in my arms; he fit perfectly in that place of a man's soul that belongs especially to a father's child. After several minutes of crying over Chance, I noticed a package sitting on the chair of his room.

The note on the package read: "To Daddy, from Chance." Inside the package I found a long-sleeved jean shirt with The Children's Hospital logo embroidered on it—a perfect gift for a perfect birthday. I locked eyes with Marti and held her gaze, the sounds and voices around me muted as my vision tunneled toward my loving wife. I barely heard what was said next:

We'll remove the central catheter this afternoon.

Huh?

And the dialysis tubes will come out tomorrow.

Are you sure? That quick?

Yes, that quick. He can go home on Thursday.

Are you sure? Thursday?

We're sure. Congratulations…and happy birthday.

The nightmare had ended, and it was all over but the celebration. Friends and doctors stopped by throughout the day to offer their best wishes, including Dr. Stanga and Dr. Fitzgerald, who had heard about our news through the staff grapevine. They were so pleased to learn that we were making arrangements to return home instead of making arrangements for long-term dialysis.

It was over.

I went to the chapel for the last time later that evening. As I sat in my usual second row seat, I thanked God for our miracle. I thanked him for the strength he had bestowed on Marti and me and, most importantly, our son Chance. I said prayers of thanks to all those who had helped us get through my son's illness. Finally, I blew a kiss to the spirits of my relatives that I had prayed to the first day.

Thanks, Gran Gran and Grandma Rossie. We did it…we did it! Thanks Grandpa Ray and Grandma Ginnie; we're going home. Thanks, Larry.

When I pulled into the garage on returning home, I realized that my perfect birthday was not yet over. My daughter Shannon had one more surprise for me. Starting with the garage door, she had left a trail of clues for me to follow inside the house. The trail included notes and pictures of Chance and the family. It led me to my office, where I saw a birthday cake sitting on my desk next to my computer screen.

Shannon had changed the picture on my screen to the one of Chance in his orange T-shirt taken two weeks before he got sick. It was my favorite picture, the one we used for our message board on the Children's website. After a day of feeling like I was near to collapsing from joy, I finally allowed myself to do so. I fell into my office chair with a *thunk* and slouched there. Tears flowed unchecked down my face once more.

The note on the cake read: "To the best dad ever: Happy Birthday! Hope you like the picture."

I ate a very big piece of cake.

THE sun had risen over our nightmare and dissipated the darkness just as quickly as the terror of illness had descended on us. Events of joy and planning and anticipation occurred at a dizzying pace, and I was giddy. We all were.

When the sun rose on Wednesday, August 31, I began preparing for my son's homecoming party. I didn't need to plan it; we had done that already the night we thought he was going to die. I just needed to execute the celebration the way we had envisioned it.

Shannon constructed a thank-you card with Chance's picture on it for the nurses on the fourth floor. She and the other kids also made a large banner to hang over our garage. My neighbor Craig and I hung it that afternoon. I looked up and stared at it for the longest time when we finished, standing in the middle of the driveway and crying, letting the hot Colorado sun warm the tears as they fell off my face. I had flashbacks to the night Chance stopped breathing, when Marti and I planned the party that we now had the privilege of holding.

Craig cried, too. He was there for us the whole time—he knew. He stood nearby and let me have my moment. Then, he said softly, "They're coming home."

Yes, they were coming home.

THE next day, Thursday, September 1, I made my last drive to the hospital. My parents joined me to help carry home a multitude of balloons, flowers, and cards and to share the moment. After delivering the thank-you card to the nurse's lounge, we said goodbye to many of the staff. Our goodbyes with the nurses were heartfelt and poignant. They were so crucial to providing nurturing care to Chance during his stay.

Chance received his last red wagon ride—his ride out of The Children's Hospital. When we got to the main doors, I asked everybody to wait. My family looked at my quizzically, as if to say, *What's the hold up, Kip? Haven't we spent enough time here?*

This moment had to be right. I knew this was going to be the biggest moment of my life. Whether that other secret miracle really happened or not didn't matter in that instant. I had been nurturing a dream in my mind's eye for three weeks that I was going to carry Chance out of that place, and I wasn't going to let any red wagon protocol get in my way!

So I picked him up and carried him out the door just like my vision in the chapel. I felt the soft, tender warmth of my son's body in my arms and realized that it had come true. God did not let me down; he blessed me with the best moment of my life. My heart sang for joy. My son's words to me from my original vision rang out over and over in my head: *Let's go, Dad!*

Let's go, Chance!

Was I dreaming? Not this time.

Marti, Chance, and I were driving home in our minivan. Driving where? Chance sat in the middle row, in his car seat.

"Oooh, Mom!" Chance exclaimed.

The Front Range foothills grew bigger in our windshield, their hazy, brown shapes inviting us onward. Table Mountain loomed large to the north.

"Mom! House, tree, hill..."

Leaving downtown Denver behind us, cars, houses, and overpasses whizzed by us on the Sixth Avenue Freeway.

"Mom! Car, bridge, building! Oooh!"

Chance was so excited, pointing out everything he saw like it was his first car ride ever—first one in a month, anyway. Table Mountain! We were going home. We were taking Chance home from the hospital.

"Oooh, Mom!"

Was I dreaming? I was not. We were home.

WHEN Marti and I thought our son was going to die, instead of planning for the worst, we planned a party. Instead of retreating into our own dark, foreboding places of terror, we held on to each other. While doctors worked to restore life-giving breath to my son, my wife and I held each other close, nose-to-nose, eye-to-eye, and celebrated Chance's recovery instead of mourning his loss. We looked forward to the best party ever: streamers, crepe paper, white cake with chocolate icing, balloons, and signs of love and welcome everywhere. We would invite the whole neighborhood.

We faced the worst and did the best we could, and it was enough; the party occurred just like we said it would.

I had so much to say before cutting the cake with the chocolate icing on Saturday, September 3. I had many people to thank for helping us get through our terrible time: friends, neighbors—my parents. Then, I turned my attention to Marti, but in front of around sixty people I completely broke down. Countless times I've given public speeches all over the country—being in front of a crowd doesn't bother me. But in front of my friends and family, with my emotions still raw from our experience, I could barely get any words out past my tears.

All I wanted to do was tell my wife how much I loved her, and that I thought she was the strongest person I knew. I had trouble with my words that day, but my tears said it all. Her eyes looked moist, too, and she smiled. But I wonder if she really knows, or really understands? Here is my opportunity to say it again:

"Your sacrifice was immeasurable, Marti; you are Chance's lifeline. You saved him, and you saved me. I love you."

We had two grand parties in five days: both celebrating renewals—the renewal of my faith and the restoration of Chance's health. The joy will last a lifetime; the celebration will never end.

I bet they had a party in heaven, too; let a thousand voices sing out—my son's second chance on life had begun.

CHAPTER 19

A Mother Speaks

Chance's mother, Marti, tells her side of the story in her own voice.

IF you want to learn to appreciate life, hang out with a five-year-old boy who knows he almost died. My son Chance shows his appreciation for life by cramming as much fun as he can into each day. He lives in the moment, observing and commenting on everything he sees. Adults could learn from him; I wish I could be like him, but being around him is enough. It's exhausting and exhilarating at the same time. Learn to appreciate life like a five-year-old—my five-year-old.

For example, bedtime is never just bedtime with Chance; it's a major event that he plans to the nth degree. Bedtime excites him as much as life does.

"Mommy, here is what we are going to do: we're going to go in the hot tub; then we're going to have my snack; then we're going to cuddle with Daddy on the couch and watch TV; then we're going upstairs; then we're going to read a story, and I want a really long story; then you are going to sing me songs; then you're going to rub my back; and you're going to rub my back for seven minutes, not five minutes; and then, I'm going to sleep."

Phew! Okay, son.

I love both my children, Loryn and Chance. I love them both so much. I love Kip's children, Shannon and TJ, too. All four of them are ours. Can you blame me, though, for possessing an extra measure of gratitude for Chance? I am utterly grateful for him, because he almost left us.

He is all boy, my goofy five year old with the crazy funny hair. You know that look a boy gets on his face that says, "I'm about to do something, and there is nothing you can do about it"? I think Chance wears that look permanently. He's always into mischief, always pushing the envelope. I adore every precious minute.

Turn your back on him and he's jumping on the couch, jumping on the bed, or climbing on the kitchen counter; you know—sword this, punch that, shoot everything in sight. It's only a matter of time before my leather couch will sport Chance's black marker artwork. He's probably dialed every number stored in my Blackberry at least once. Blink your eyes and he will destroy your house. I love every minute.

I'll always be very protective of him. I almost lost him once, and I won't let that happen again. I refuse to let Chance eat beef in restaurants. I know the possibility of it happening a second time is small, but I'm not taking that risk. I don't think he would survive it again. Chance got sick and almost died once because of food he ate that we willingly gave him. Never again.

"I'm allergic to 'hangaber,'" he says.

No kidding.

GIVING an eighteen-month-old child with failed kidneys two doses of morphine is a bad, bad idea. Take it from me.

After Chance's surgery to place the dialysis tubes in his tummy, he went downhill fast. As usual, I lay underneath him in his bed after the surgery. He would often lie on my lap in the hospital, even with all the tubes and things sticking out from him. It was the only way I knew to keep him calm. It reminded me of the day the doctors placed him on top of me after he was born.

He really was going downhill fast, getting more and more restless. His stomach became distended, and it bloated up in front of my eyes. He began to wheeze as his breathing became more labored. Something was not right. I told our nurse my concerns several times, but she said Chance was just experiencing normal post-operative symptoms.

That explanation just didn't work for me. My instincts told me something was not right. I looked past the nurse and told Kip to get the doctor. I only trusted Kip. He is not fine—*get the doctor.*

Kip returned alone. Dr. Fitzgerald was in the break room, he said; he didn't want to disturb her.

Something is wrong.

What?

I don't know, but there's something wrong.

Just as I said that, my son stopped breathing. He was looking me in the eyes when he just gasped and stopped breathing. *Go get the doctor, now!*

Thank God Kip was there. I needed him in that moment more than ever. I had no idea what to do. Kip left again, this time sprinting down the hallway to retrieve Dr. Fitzgerald. After he left I stood up still holding Chance. *What do I do?*

Dr. Fitzgerald had an incredulous look on her face when she entered the room. The last report she had heard from the duty nurse was that Chance was resting comfortably after surgery.

Not really.

He's not breathing! What's wrong? What's wrong?

Dr. Fitzgerald stood there, amazed.

Do something!

She just stood there and looked at me. I wanted to scream. I was screaming—on the inside. Chance was turning blue. I held him out to the doctor to show her his blue face.

Do something. Won't you do something? This is my son. Please...

My eyes started to tear up with frustration. My son was slipping away in my arms and nobody would do anything. After everything he had already been through, were we going to lose him then?

What I didn't know at the time was that Dr. Fitzgerald really was doing something. Her mind was spinning through the scenario, trying to put the pieces together. Her surprised face changed in an instant to one of action that said, "I've got him." When she spoke, she did so with authority to bark out a series of orders: *I need oxygen, an intubation kit, X-ray...STAT!*

Then my turn came to look dumbfounded. A flock of hospital personnel descended on our room with a rush. I looked on in shock and amazement as they mobilized around me, but I continued to hold Chance until Molly entered the room and took him from me. I couldn't bear to let go but I realized I was just getting in the way. I'll never forget the look on my baby's gasping face when I gave him up.

Molly told me to go find Kip outside. I left the room on trembling legs; I could barely walk. *Kip? Where are you? I need you. I can't do this anymore.* My knees buckled and I nearly fell down. Kip caught me and led me to a place to sit in the waiting room.

He's not breathing...he's going to die! We're going to lose him...

Kip took over and saved me from my despair. He said no, absolutely not. While we waited, he told me about the great big party we were going to throw Chance the day we took him home from the hospital. We planned that party for forty-five minutes. It was going to be the best party ever: streamers, crepe paper, white cake with chocolate icing, balloons, and signs of love and welcome everywhere. We would invite the whole neighborhood.

KIP beats himself up about how he handled Chance's illness in the first few days. I wish he would stop. What delays? He only let one bloody stool pass without taking action, by my count. I'm the one who denied the seriousness of the situation, for quite a while, in fact. I kept thinking Chance only had the flu. If it weren't for Kip's insistence, we would not have sought the medical attention we did, when we did. Thank God! He saved Chance's life.

I couldn't have made it through without Kip. All I knew was that I had to hold my son, or else. Chance and I needed an advocate, someone to be a bulldog with doctors and nurses on our behalf. I needed someone to take care of our household, to pay the bills, feed the dogs, and to notify our friends and family about what was happening. Kip was that person.

Kip kept our lives functional while I spent all those days in the hospital. He remembered birthdays, anniversaries, and even our son TJ's soccer match. I would have forgotten to eat and sleep without him. I needed him. He never forgot we had a marriage that required nurturing if we were to function as partners.

When my darkest hour came and I found myself asking if we were fighting too hard for something that was not meant to be, Kip saved me a second time by sharing with me the vision he saw as a result of his unceasing prayers for Chance's recovery. I had witnessed enough of my child's pain. I couldn't take anymore, but Kip would not let me give up. He told me Chance would leave the hospital someday and described to me exactly how we would carry our son out the door.

I believed him.

DOES a young child remember pain? I ask myself that every time Chance touches the scars on his tummy. I wince when he does. How much? I wish *I* didn't have to remember. Nothing pierces a mother's heart more than hearing her son scream from a pain that he doesn't understand and can't verbalize for hours and hours, day after day. I pray to God he remembers nothing of the pain.

You never know, though. When your son tells his pediatrician that she "saved his life" you never know. It wounds a mother's soul to remember. I pray to God that *he* doesn't.

I don't think Chance slept the entire time he was on dialysis at The Children's Hospital. For ten or more hours each night that machine would cycle every twenty minutes, swishing fluid around in his tummy, then draining it back out. Those fluids rushing through him had to be uncomfortable. Sometimes the machine would malfunction. What happened? Where did the cycle stop: fluid in or fluid out? Where was the dialysis nurse? He never slept, and neither did I.

The incisions on his stomach that allowed the tubes to enter and exit his body were probably the most painful things to him. They were packed in open wounds that required constant cleaning to avoid infection. Chance knew when the nurses planned to clean his incisions. He screamed so loud I'm sure the whole floor heard him. His screams echoed around that entire hospital. A mom can only take so much.

Dialysis was not his only source of agony. Catheters, IVs, heart monitors, PICC lines, needles, dialysis tubes, gastric tubes, intubation tubes, tubes—tubes—tubes—it went on and on. Diarrhea, vomiting, seizures, cramps, bloating, inflammation, anemia, extreme irritability, sleeplessness…how much could the spirit of a child not yet two years old endure? What about me? I swear I felt everything he did. My anguish for his sake was unbearable; it constricted my gut like a vice and threatened to turn me inside out, as if I had a physical disease of my own.

On top of all that, we were so worried that Chance would never regain the use of his kidneys. We dreaded that possibility, because Chance was too young at the time for a kidney transplant. If he survived but his kidneys did not, that meant two to three years of that horrible dialysis until he was big enough for the transplant list. Three years of those awful tubes in his tummy; three years of being hooked up to that machine each night. We despaired to think of all the things we were going to have to give up: sports, traveling, daycare…what would our lives be like—infections, complications, and unending sleeplessness?

We would have done it, of course. We would have endured. We would have done anything for him. What about a kidney transplant, though? It's a risky operation for adults, even more so for kids—I looked it up. It didn't matter because he hadn't survived his infection, yet. We were still in the hospital fighting for his life.

This horrible infection left Chance unrecognizable, a dim reflection of his former physical and emotional self. He didn't even have the desire to put his thumb in his mouth. What if the continuation of dialysis for three more years continued to suck away his personality as much as it sucked toxin-filled fluids out of his body? I wanted my son back desperately.

Suck your thumb, Chance. Please. I want my son back. Please suck your thumb!

WHEN the E. coli toxins finally subsided, he began to lose his irritability, and the dialysis finally began balancing his metabolism. We then started taking trips outside his room in a red wagon. The Children's Hospital had wheelchairs, but most kids wanted to ride around in those red wagons. They were everywhere. I loaded Chance up in his red wagon, and I pulled him around the hospital and the grounds. He loved to go outside to sit in the sunshine.

The Children's Hospital also had a wacky kinetic motion sculpture of these balls racing around a maze. It's hard to describe. Chance loved it. We would stare at it for half an hour at a time. I think it soothed him, made him feel better by causing him to forget the pain.

Besides his red wagon trips, Chance and I had a daily ritual of reading a special book. Chance bugged me to read it to him every day. It was called *What Do Toddlers Do?* I don't remember where it came from. Somebody brought it from home, or it was a gift…whatever.

The book was full of pictures of kids Chance's age doing things kids like to do: swinging, swimming, eating ice cream. Every day he wanted me to read that book—and not just once, but over and over. I told him that he was going to do those things when he got out of the hospital. I could tell that's what he was thinking, too. That's why he wanted me to read it to him. He knew then what toddlers should do, just as he knows now what boys should do. He lives life to the fullest, my brave little man. He wasn't going to give up.

Read books—sing songs—play rock-paper-scissors—look at the trees—watch TV....

Got it!

Jump on the bed—dive off the counter—torment the dog—draw on the couch....

Not so fast!

Have fun—live life like a five-year-old.

CHAPTER 20

Second Chance

"If we couldn't laugh, we would all go insane."

—JIMMY BUFFETT

MARTI and I needed a change in latitude after five stressful, fear-filled weeks dealing with Chance's illnesses at The Children's Hospital. Yes, *illnesses*. Just two days after our triumphant welcome home party, we found ourselves back in a room on the fourth floor of that institution with him. Our stay this time came courtesy of a C. diff infection.

Life is not as tidy as we like it to be sometimes; sometimes, it just gets messy. Just when we thought we were home free and on the road to health with Chance, another setback occurred. Like the first time, though, we rallied together and we survived.

Our nurse friends on that floor were just as dismayed to see us return as we were to be there. *Clostridium difficile* is another intestinal bacterium that can cause...severe diarrhea, of course. Chance was frantic most of the time; his memories of his first stay were still quite vivid, obviously. However, this time the illness was much easier to diagnose, treatable, and self-limiting; we were home again in four days.

A few weeks later, Marti and I treated ourselves to a weekend getaway to Las Vegas. We needed to let off some steam and reconnect with each other. I usually go to Vegas each March to enjoy the NCAA tournament with a friend of mine. Jimmy Buffett's Margaritaville is one of our favorite hangouts, because we like the music. So that was the first place I thought of to take Marti once we arrived. As we sat in that loud, energetic lounge with fake palm trees and a large sea plane hanging from the ceiling, our pent up stress began to melt away. We felt very close to each other.

I didn't plan on telling Marti my secrets that night, but as the evening progressed and we became more relaxed, my defenses evaporated. Over a cheeseburger in paradise, I told her everything I had been holding back about my activities during our stay at The Children's Hospital. I told her about my daily trips to the chapel. I shared with her about my prayers, who I prayed to, and all the details about my vision and how I meditated on it every single day. Finally, I told her that I prayed for a miracle. I told her that I believed we received one and described what I saw the night I stayed with Chance in his room.

I felt so nervous that Marti wasn't going to believe me that I preceded my speech with a disclaimer that she was going to think I was crazy. I laid it all out there for Marti to process and digest. "What do you think of me, now?" I asked.

She gave me the opposite reaction. She broke down, cried, and said she believed me. She told me that she had been wondering why Chance recovered, since there seemed to be no medical explanation. Now she knew. I had given her the explanation she had been looking for.

Then there were no more secrets between us, and our joy in the moment was complete. We laughed and began enjoying our

Las Vegas getaway in earnest. Jimmy Buffett was right: if we couldn't laugh, then we would all go insane.

The rest of the weekend was a whirlwind of swimming pools, luxurious accommodations, shows, and fine dining. We felt whole once again. We had a chance to restore the romance and adventure of our lives. We attended the Cirque du Soleil show *O* and took in a Barry Manilow concert. You know I am a feeler.

LIFE returned to normal for us after that. The slow, agonizing crisis was over, and time sped up to its normal pace once more. Too fast, maybe. Milestones come and go at an alarming rate. I relish them all and cherish them in my heart, except for my own birthdays, perhaps. They are bittersweet for me each year. The feelings of guilt and self-blame I still feel for Chance's sake become intensified each birthday that passes. I get clingy with Chance on my birthdays, like he might be going somewhere, and I'll never get him back. My birthday is almost indistinguishable from my memories of his illness in my mind.

I don't know why I blame myself so much for Chance getting sick. The guilt doesn't make sense, but it's still there. Healing is a slow process. I don't know what I could have done differently. Once he got sick I did the best I could, and he survived. Guilt is an insidious thing, though, it's hard to completely banish from your life. I learned how to ask God for miracles. Now I need to learn how to ask for forgiveness. Whom do I ask? God…Marti…Chance?

The facility we knew as The Children's Hospital is closed and boarded up now. They moved the main hospital to another location in a suburb a few years ago. I don't know what they are going to do with the old building, but I hope they tear it down.

Maybe my guilt will crumble down with it. I doubt it; it's just a building. My feelings of remorse are more real than a collection of bricks and glass. Whom do I ask?

Will you forgive me, Chance?

WE have been blessed with many opportunities to share our story with the media, contributing to the awareness of food borne illnesses. Our message is simple: be aware, be vigilant; the consequences can be deadly. ABC's Nightline interviewed me for a segment on the Food Safety Conference that was hosted in Denver one year. Colorado congresswoman Dianna DeGette introduced some food-safety initiatives and asked me to participate in a news conference with her. When the local media heard what we were up to, they interviewed us for the nightly news. The ABC station taped Marti and me in our living room with Chance running laps around the couch, pushing his stroller. Later, up in my office, the NBC affiliate taped Chance and me for another interview. While I was answering questions for them, he kept pulling up his shirt to show off his dialysis scars.

Chance himself is learning to pray. He is ahead of the curve in that regard; I hope he keeps this practice up the rest of his life. His prayers are amusing but tender and heartfelt. There is something about the guileless, noble prayers of a child that I find very endearing. He is in charge of saying grace around our dinner table and is very serious about it. Everyone must be in their place first.

I can't help but peek over my folded hands around the table as Chance waits for his cue. My family is by far the very best part of me. Shannon, nineteen, is finishing her freshman year at Colorado University. She studies English and theatre arts education and pledged the Tri-Delta sorority. TJ is nearing the end of his first year at Golden High School, earning honors. He still plays soccer but has found a new interest in long-distance track events; he is fifteen. Loryn just turned twelve and continues to cultivate her performance career. She recently participated in a production of *The Sound of Music* at a local theatre company.

Finally, I'll steal a glance at my soul mate, Marti—the mother of these wonderful children and the rock that supports our family. Chance and I honored what she means to us by making a bracelet out of the rock that the mysterious Father Anderson gave me in the hospital. We gave it to her on Mother's Day, 2006 and included the Bible verse that meant so much to me at the time, Psalm 62. She still wears the bracelet proudly when she can.

I know that she would do whatever she could to take care of any one of these children around our dinner table, just as she took care of Chance.

I have a fabulous family, and of course Chance is in charge. When everyone is seated around the table to his satisfaction, but not until everyone is served, he'll begin his prayer. *Dear Jesus: Thank-you for this food. Help Miss Kay, help Grandpa and Misty to feel better, please take care of Susie, and help Daddy's owie heal.* The prayers of a child: always other people first. He then pauses for a long time, making sure he's got everything covered. Then, he'll finish with a rapid flourish: *In Jesus' name, Amen.*

IT'S after supper now, and *American Idol* is playing on TV. Chance and I are on the couch eating potato chips. Marti joins us this night. We surround our son like book-ends, wrapping him in love. We have the animal kingdom with us: Chance's treasured collection of Beanie Babies. We have Aslan, the Lion; Sasha, the other lion; Spot the dog; and Stripes, the tiger. Tonight we have a new addition: a rattlesnake. Nobody knows what its name is.

He's the boy with a plan, our young son. He has his goals for the summer already laid out: he is going to learn to swim and ride his bike without training wheels. I'm guessing he will achieve both by the end of June. He is making the most of his second chance on life.

The potato chips are finished, and he puts his thumb in his mouth. Then, he yanks it out again. A few minutes later it's back in his mouth. Marti and I look over his head at each other, wink, and smile. We adore him when he sucks his thumb, but it is probably a good thing he is trying to quit. Thumb sucking is not the most sanitary thing for a boy who's in daycare and almost ready for school. We nearly lost him to a severe, food-borne illness, and we'll do whatever it takes to keep him safe now, to see him grow and thrive.

Besides, he knows he's getting older, and thumb sucking is not dignified for a school boy. "I'm going to start Kindergarten soon," he says. Tell me about it—I'll miss you when you are there.

My miracle boy is growing up.

WEEKS passed before I could muster the courage to tell Marti what I saw in Chance's room that climactic night at The Children's Hospital. An even longer time passed before I could bring myself to tell someone outside our family. I felt self-conscious, convinced people would think I was some sort of religious nut. I'm not, and neither am I prone to hallucinations or radical departures from reality. I'm not trying to force anyone to believe in

God or miracles; I'm simply telling the truth of my experience as I saw it. I wasn't a believer in miracles before, but now I am.

One thing I learned is that God does indeed work in miraculous ways here on earth. He chooses to work in the lives of ordinary people like me, even those of us with conflicted ideas of faith. Marti and I feel that God had a plan for Chance and our family. It's part of God's plan for us that he recovered. We don't know why God chose us for this miracle; we just know that he did. Now, we have the opportunity to find out what that plan was—maybe it's to help other parents going through the same things we went through. Maybe it's to provide encouragement to people who don't believe in miracles. All we know is that someone touched Chance that night, and it wasn't a nurse or a doctor. We also know that there is no medical reason why he suddenly began to improve. Parents need the courage to hope for miracles. I know one thing—Marti wasn't a believer before, but she is now.

So what did I see that night in Chance's room? I had my doubts at first, as I've said, but I think Chance knew the answer all along. I remember the first time I told this aspect of his tale to someone else; Chance sat with us at a restaurant with friends when I did. He was busting to help me tell the story.

"A slight noise woke me up around two in the morning. I saw a faint light on the other side of the curtain; I couldn't tell what it was."

Dad?

"I pulled the curtain back and saw what I thought was a nurse standing in profile by Chance's bedside. Who was it?"

Dad?

"I rubbed the sleep out of my eyes and looked again. The figure had a hazy outline, sort of a glow to it, and it extended its hands over Chance's chest. I couldn't tell who or what it was."

Hey, Dad!

"I pinched myself in the arms to make sure I was awake. I definitely wasn't dreaming but I was paralyzed, unable to speak or rise."

I know what it was, Dad!

"I gasped when I realized the thing wasn't even touching the floor, it was completely *hovering* over my son. The glow got more intense the closer it got to Chance. I couldn't believe what I was seeing. It looked like it touched Chance's stomach, near his incisions."

Dad...Dad, Dad!

"And then, in an instant, the vision was gone, and the room returned to blackness. I felt chills all over my body and I began to tremble. I kept thinking, what was that?"

Dad, it was my Angel!

Your angel?

Yes, you're right, son. Don't ever forget that you have an angel watching over you.

God is "cheating" for you, too.

EPILOGUE

MY son Chance continues to be a healthy, active boy to this day. I have so much to look forward to as a father to all our children, and my gratitude in knowing that Chance will always be among them is immeasurable. We'll be able to spend thousands of nights watching TV on the couch together as buddies—father and son.

We don't know precisely how well Chance's kidneys are functioning. He continues to have protein detected in his urine, so we suspect they are not 100 percent. Not ideal, but he can live with them at their current level. The need for a kidney transplant diminishes as time goes on and he gets stronger and older. His immune system is not the best; it seems like we are always fighting off a cold. His tummy is still slightly distended, but we expect that to disappear as he grows, too. His scars will remain forever.

Marti and I are blessed, because we have experienced grace in a huge way. When I hear about other children who have died from HUS or lost the use of their kidneys, I feel their pain. I know that would be us too, if not for the grace of God. I don't know why Chance was touched by God, but I feel lucky and blessed that he was. I have to blink and rub my eyes to remind myself that this sandy-haired kid is really here—body, soul, and potential intact. I don't know what the future holds for my son, but I am already confident he will make the most of this second chance he has been given in life.

I have learned so much since that fateful month of August, 2005. I learned about the strength of a family, the love of a wife and mother, the power of prayer, and the will to live of a brave, small boy. I also discovered fortitude within me, which I didn't know existed, and found a sincere desire to offer hope to parents who face similar dark days of a child's illness. I will continue to be a public voice, as long as the spirit leads me, encouraging parents to be cautious about the safety of the food they give their children. I hope that someday no family has to experience what we did, ever again.

Children are so resilient, but when they are ill they need their parents to be strong for them. When I thought my strength had departed without possibility of recall, a courageous nurse took a risk and told me that my son would not die at a time when only God knew what the outcome would be. The surge of confidence I felt in that moment was a gift sent from heaven.

I can never repay her fully; I wish I remembered her name, but I don't. Instead, I'll pay her forward by offering this story to parents of sick children everywhere. This is my gift to them—a shot of confidence in the arm, if they need one.

You can fight for your children, no matter what happens. You have the strength within you. When you think all is lost, remember the words that the nurse spoke to me in my darkest hour; recall the hope they contain; then, say a prayer and leave the rest to God.

"We do NOT let kids die of E. coli at The Children's Hospital."

Amen.

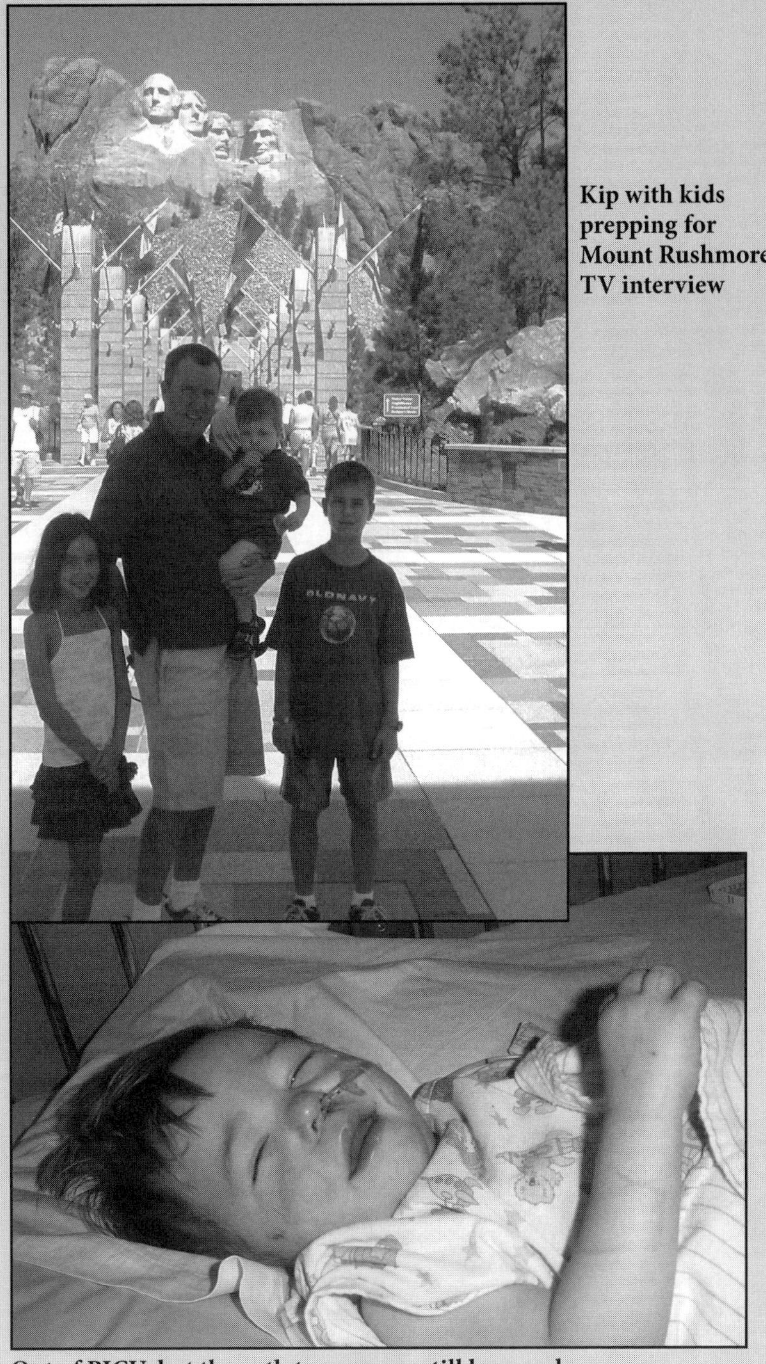

Kip with kids prepping for Mount Rushmore TV interview

Out of PICU, but the path to recovery still long and fraught with crisis

Molly proudly displaying Marti's anniversary gift to Kip—photo of urine taken with the mystery Polaroid camera

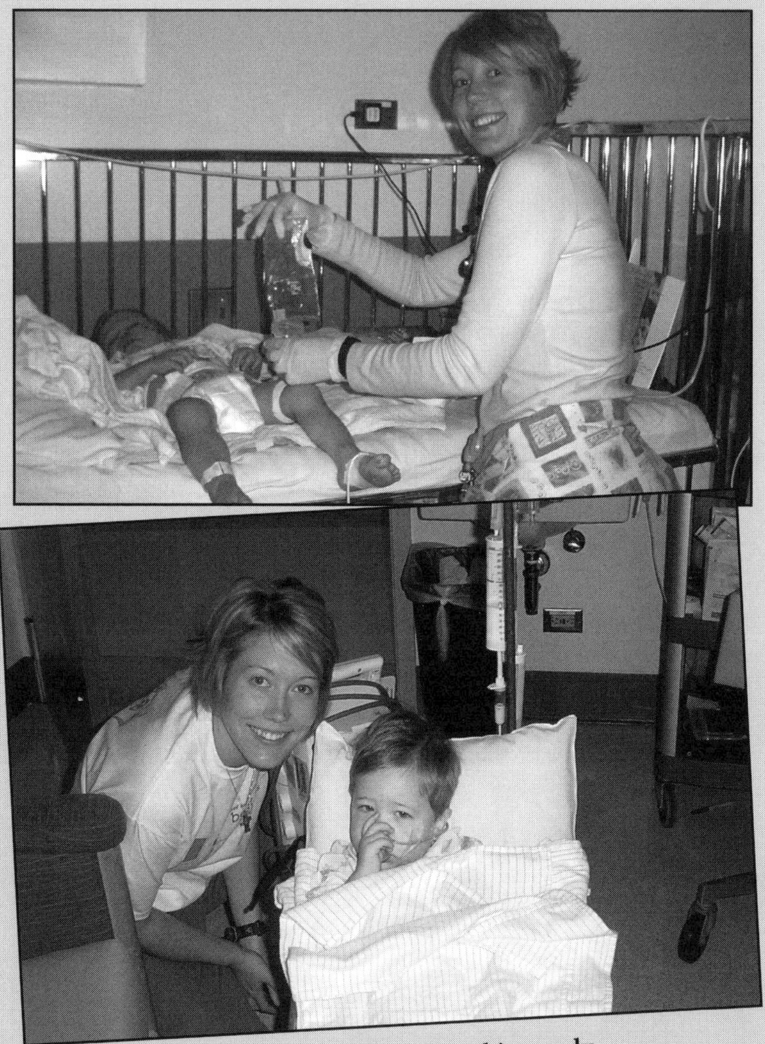

Molly posing with Chance after getting him ready for his first red wagon ride

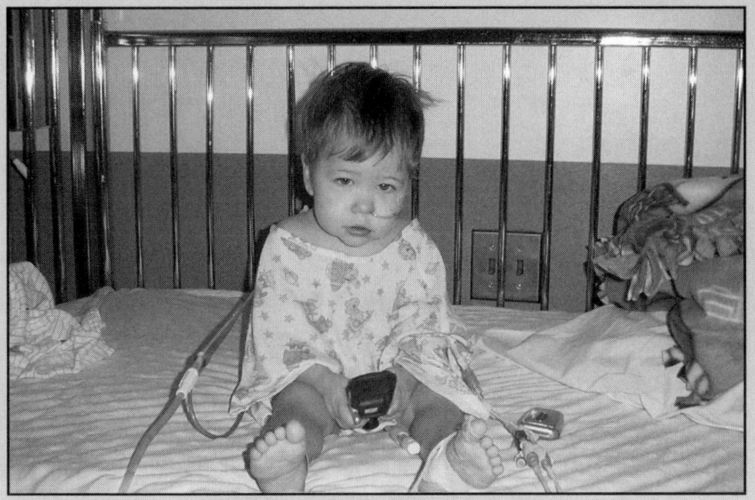

Chance dialing every number in Marti's Blackberry

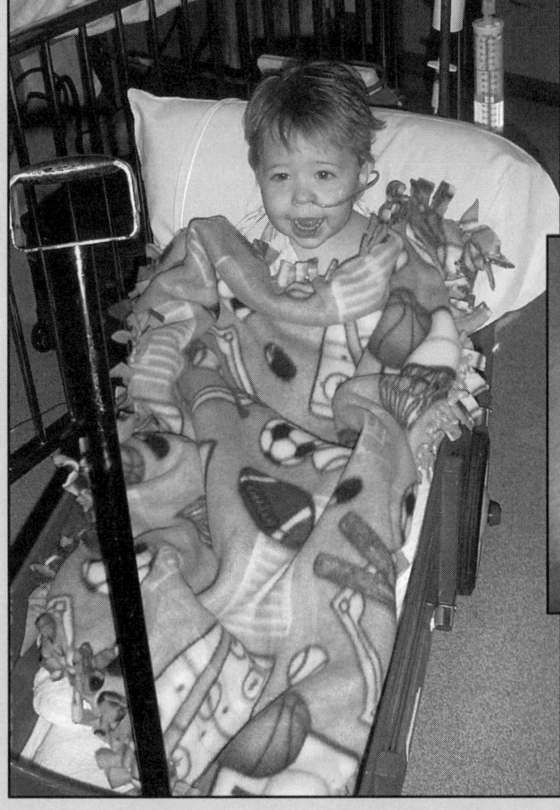

Chance enjoying his daily red wagon ride

The bracelet made from the rock given to Kip by the mysterious Father Anderson, presented to Marti on Mother's Day 2006 by Chance

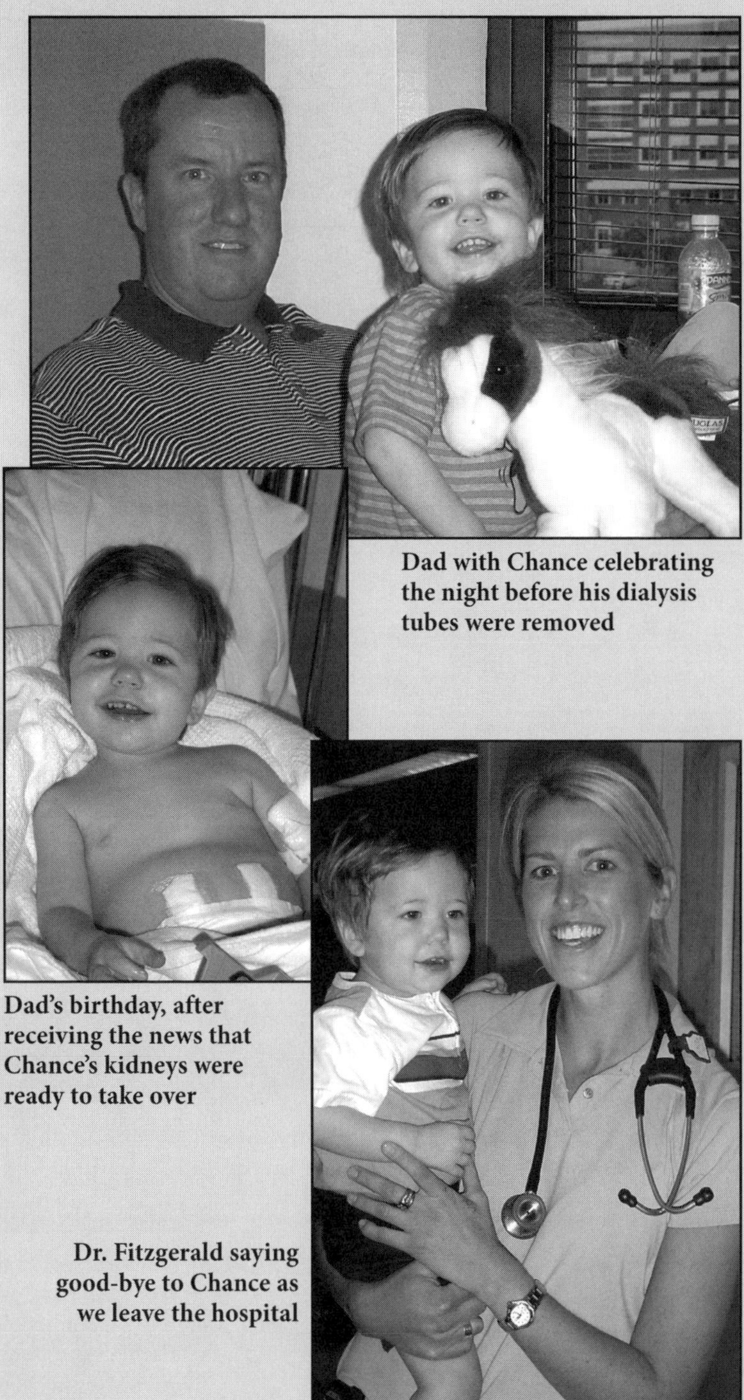

Dad with Chance celebrating the night before his dialysis tubes were removed

Dad's birthday, after receiving the news that Chance's kidneys were ready to take over

Dr. Fitzgerald saying good-bye to Chance as we leave the hospital

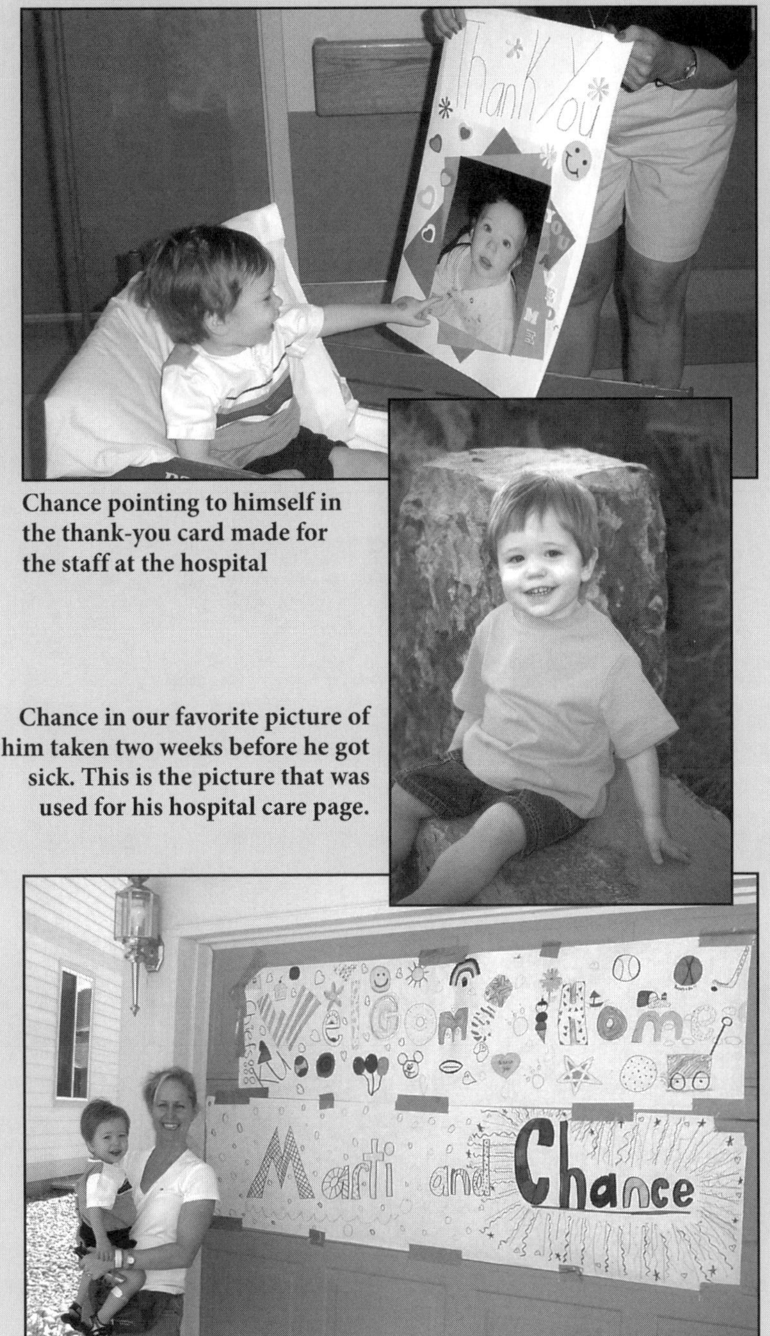

Chance pointing to himself in the thank-you card made for the staff at the hospital

Chance in our favorite picture of him taken two weeks before he got sick. This is the picture that was used for his hospital care page.

Marti and Chance admiring the welcome home banner hung by Kip and Craig, our neighbor

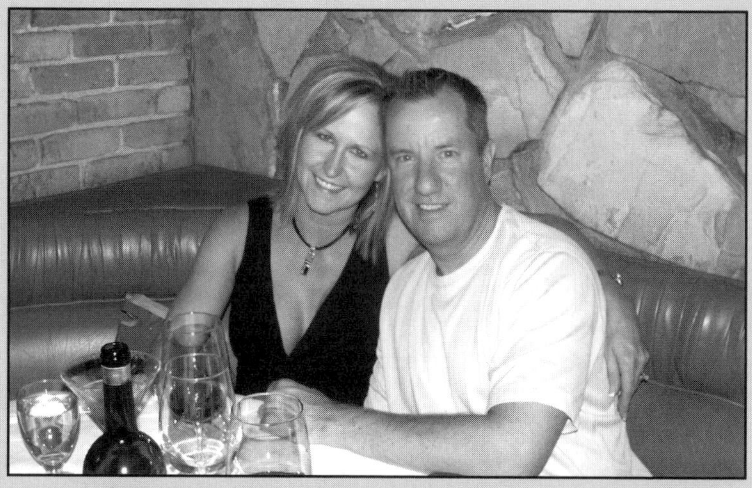

Marti and Kip in Las Vegas celebrating Chance's recovery

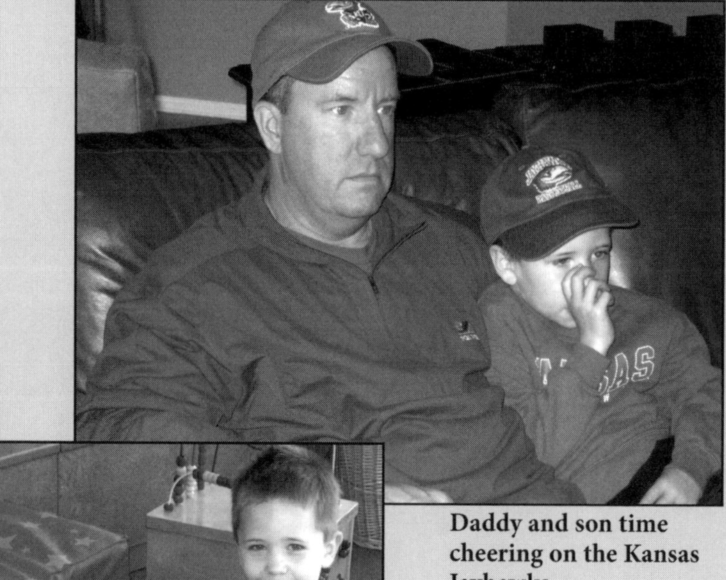

Daddy and son time cheering on the Kansas Jayhawks

Recent picture of our speed-racer revving his engine

ABOUT THE AUTHOR

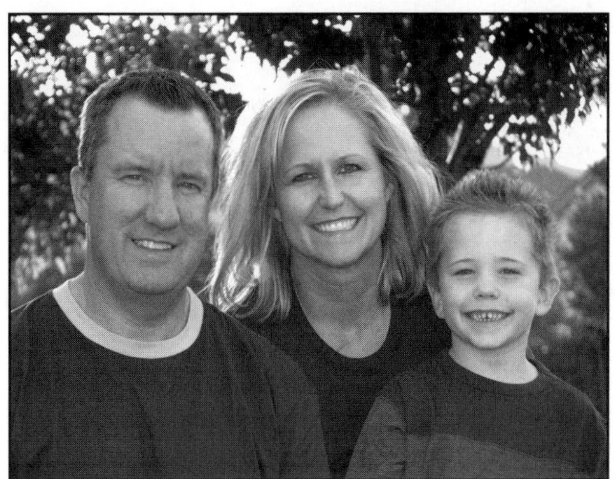

Kip, Marti, and Chance

KIP MOORE lives in Golden, Colorado, with his wife, Marti, and their four children, Shannon, TJ, Loryn, and Chance. They share their poignant story in the hope of saving just one family from the pain and fear they endured.

Give the Gift of

Second Chance

The Story of a Father's Faith, a Mother's Strength, and a Child's Will to Live

to Your Friends and Colleagues

CHECK YOUR LEADING BOOKSTORE OR ORDER HERE

❑ **YES**, I want _____ copies of ***Second Chance*** at $17.95 each, plus $4.95 shipping per book (Colorado residents please add 52¢ sales tax per book). Canadian orders must be accompanied by a postal money order in U.S. funds. Allow 15 days for delivery.

My check or money order for $__________ is enclosed.

Please charge my: ❑ Visa ❑ MasterCard ❑ Discover ❑ American Express

Name ______________________________

Organization ______________________________

Address ______________________________

City/State/Zip ______________________________

Phone ______________ Email ______________

Card # ______________________________

Exp. Date __________ Signature ______________

Please make your check payable and return to:

Second Chance Publishing LLC

5587 Dunraven Lane • Golden, CO 80403

Call your credit card order to: 720-560-9912

Order online at: www.secondchancestory.com

kip@secondchancestory.com